Tomorrow's

Technology Today

Creating the State of the Art Dental Office

Because Your Patients (and Your Team Members)

Expect Nothing Less

By James W. Rotondo

Acknowledgements

This book has been underway for quite a while now. As a long-time member of the dental community, I have drawn from my extensive experience over the years to contribute to this book.

I would like to acknowledge the countless clients across southern California (and across the country) who have allowed me the opportunity to work with their offices and staff members to help build a more positive environment. I spent many hours simply watching the inner dynamics of some of the most successful dental practices, as well as and some of the worst.

I could not have written this book without help from such a large, diverse, and intelligent group of professionals.

I'd also like to thank my wife and friends who have continuously read and re-read this book for me.

When you set out to write a book, you have the core ideas, and you have the knowledge of how to write words on paper.

This experience has taught me that you cannot do it alone, and I was very fortunate to have Michael Levin of BusinessGhost, Inc. escort me through this process. Without the support of Michael and his staff, this book would have never been published.

If you own your own practice, perhaps this book can serve as guidance as to how technology can affect your office.

I hope you find useful ideas within these pages. I wrote this book as a means to put down on paper what I spend my days discussing with dentists all over the country. I'd love to hear your story as well. Please don't hesitate to contact me. I am always happy to help.

James W. Rotondo

Contents

Chapter 1

Dr. Betty Rubble Will See You Now

Fred and Wilma Flintstone have just relocated to the town of Bedrock. Like everyone who moves to a new place, they have to find a new dentist. They look in the phone book and settle on Dr. Betty Rubble. When they arrive at her office, it feels like they have stepped back to the Stone Age of dentistry. Feelings of doubt and uncertainty cloud their senses.

In their previous hometown, the Flintstones saw a dentist whose office was completely up-to-date, from the beautiful furnishings in the waiting room to the state-of-the-art computer technology that assisted the dentist and his entire team.

Everything was high-tech, high-touch, brand-new, and well planned. Even the dental chair in which Fred or Wilma would recline during dentistry had all the latest features—headphones with a wide-screen TV positioned in just the right place. The dental chair even had heat and massage functions. They could relax and almost forget they were going to the dentist.

Dr. Rubble's office, by contrast, feels outdated and even depressing. From the time that Fred and Wilma step into the waiting room, they have a sense that things are not right. As they look around the waiting room area, their senses are again jolted. The seating in the waiting room looks a little dingy, worn out, definitely uninviting and uncomfortable. As they approach the transaction counter to check in for their appointments, they notice an old and chipped Formica countertop with a little sliding glass window that separates the receptionist at the front desk from the patients.

The young woman is operating what appears to be the only computer in the whole dental office, and, since this is Bedrock, it is not a PC.

It is a BC, which stands for "barely connected." Pretty much everything in the office, from the charts to the billing mechanism to the scheduling, is filled in by hand. Fred and Wilma announce themselves to the receptionist, and she asks them to take a seat in the waiting room. They glance at each other nervously, as if they both were unsure of the experiences they were about to have.

If the waiting area is this far behind the times, what awaits them once they get into the operatory?

The receptionist asks Fred and Wilma to come back up to the window to get forms that they will need to fill out for the doctor. Since this is their first visit to Dr. Betty Rubble, they will need to provide all the information for their charts.

Puzzled, Fred and Wilma take the forms and clipboard back to their seats. Yet another wave of insecurity comes over them. This was not the way they had gotten used to things at their previous dentist. As their concern over the paper forms increases, they become reluctant to actually fill out all the requested information. Instead they provide only the basics, leaving off things like employment questions and Social Security information.

After returning the forms to the receptionist, they're told that the doctor is running a few minutes behind and are asked if they can wait just a bit more. In reality, Dr. Rubble lacked a means of keeping track of how much time each treatment or procedure was anticipated to take. As a result, the waiting room slowly fills with other Bedrockians who are also in that same uncertain, unhappy state as Fred and Wilma. When a dental assistant finally ushers the Flintstones back to the operatory, Fred and Wilma catch a look at the dentist's desk.

It is piled almost to the ceiling with paper. How would the office ever keep track of their dental issues or histories? They glance at the floor and see old linoleum laminate tiles. There are no baseboard moldings; the tile simply wraps up the wall a few inches. From floor to ceiling the room reminds them of a clinical asylum from an old horror movie. Fred and Wilma begin to giggle as they reminisce about the movie *Little Shop of Horrors.*

Once in the operatory, they see that the dental chair is old, well-worn, and discolored. The padding is practically flat. The covering is plastic, not leather, and it looks a million years old, even by Bedrock standards.

The metal components of the chair appear rusted or oxidized, and the chair itself looks as though it is so old that it would be very hard to keep clean.

The dental equipment hardly inspires any more confidence. Much of it is discolored and tired looking. Some of the mechanical component switches are broken, and a hissing sound punctuates the room because one of the devices is leaking air. The cabinetry and the blinds are ancient. There are no computers, no monitors, no TVs, and no sound system—there are no patient comforts at all.

Fred and Wilma see a stack of twenty or more charts on the table next to the dental chair, and they realize that Dr. Rubble probably has not gotten around to completing yesterday's charts. How can she possibly remember each detail for each patient, even a day later? How could they be sure that some vital information about their dental histories, or their X-rays, or something else important, wouldn't be lost in those piles?

Worse yet, they are left alone with these charts. If so inclined they could grab a handful and begin reading about other patients' treatments.

A horrified feeling of insecurity sets in. "What happens after our visit today?" Wilma asks. "Will our charts be added to this pile right here for others to read as well?"

Finally a dental assistant enters the room and barely greets Fred and Wilma, even though they are new patients. She looks very rushed and as depressed as her surroundings.

Fred and Wilma take one look at her, look at each other, and whisper, "Let's get out of here." And yes, they do in fact leave, but not before stopping at the front desk to get their personal information back.

Patients will leave without being seen, just as in a restaurant that fails to provide good service.

Every time I visit a dental office that has not been updated for ten or twenty or even thirty years, I feel as though I have slipped back in time to the town of Bedrock. As a Dental Technology Consultant, I feel what they must feel. My senses tell me that the dental office has fallen too far behind to take proper care of me and my family.

Our organization is unique because of our client base and what we do for them.

Our Clients: We chose the dental community due to the complexity of the business. A private practice dental office has a great deal of technology versus a standard medical office, and far more technology than corporate America.

However, we discovered that the dental community was being serviced by standard IT personnel. This is not bad, just not focused.

What We Do: We provide a variety of services to the dental community beginning with the "What do I do now?" question that is asked by so many dentists stuck in yesteryear.

We are not a standard IT company, but rather an organization that provides technology consulting far beyond installing a computer. We supply the office staff with the tools they need to do better business, while helping them to create an environment appealing to their patients' senses. We coach the doctor and staff on all the whats and hows.

We meet with other support personnel such as contractors, designers, and financial planners to help the doctor build a place where they are all happy to work and proud of their establishment.

- **Sound**
- **Sight**
- **Smell**
- **Touch**
- **Taste**

Remember, we use these senses to collect and sort information so that we can help our clients make better decisions.

Our company designs and installs the state-of-the-art technology that dentists use throughout their offices, but what we really install is a sense of certainty. Certainty for the doctor—he knows that everything he needs, from the right information to the right tools, is at the touch of his fingertips, because his environment is absolutely state of the art.

Certainty for the patient—he knows, from just one look around the waiting room, the technology behind the counter, the wide-screen TV for his enjoyment, the computer technology in the operatory, and the tidy, paperless office of the dentist himself, that he is going to be well taken care of. When patients do not experience that sense of certainty, they leave for other practices where they will surely find it. When team members in the dental office do not feel that they have been given the latest and the greatest tools and technology in order to serve their patients with maximum efficiency and comfort, they leave, too … and take jobs with competing dental offices.

In this book, I will show you how to transform your office—most likely for less money than you might have imagined—into the futuristic kind of technologically-driven dental suite that inspires confidence in your patients and your team, and motivates your patients to send their friends to you and you alone. It is our job to make the lives of dentists easier.

Doctors come to us and say, "What's wrong? What do I need to change? What is going on with my office? Why aren't I retaining patients? Why aren't I getting referrals at the same rate as in the past?" Many times the answers to these questions are simple—the dental office environment and technology within that office are not where they need to be, and the dentist ends up losing business to another nicer, more updated office.

When that happens, they call us. And their needs reflect their different personalities. Some dentists like to be the forerunner, on the leading edge of technology, with an office that surpasses everyone else in their communities. In that sense, they are acutely aware of competition for the kind of patients with whom they want to work—people who show up on time, who accept treatment, and who can afford to pay for it. For these dentists, we provide total office makeovers.

Other dentists might not be interested in redoing their entire approach to technology, but they are ready to make a few changes, and measure the return on investment from those changes. Some dentists are so far behind the curve that any change we make has a drastic impact on their practice and their entire lives. For example, I recently visited a dental office where the doctor has only two chairs. He is a wonderful, older gentleman, and a fantastic dentist who has worked for many, many years.

For his office needs, we installed a new computer and new digital X-ray equipment. The moment that was the most enjoyable for us was when he said, practically with a tear in his eye, "You mean I can finally turn off my developing unit and never have to develop film again?"

"Yes," we told him.

"Oh, I hate that machine. Thank goodness. I am never buying developer solutions and film ever again. I am just going digital."

I know he is going to call us back in six months and say, "I am ready for another piece. What do we do next?" And we'll be there to deliver the next piece of technology for him.

So that is an example of a dentist who was in dire need of the benefits that state-of-the-art technology can provide. Most dentists are considerably further along the curve than this gentleman, though. I recently met with a doctor who wanted to go paperless. "Great, we'll get it handled for you," I told him.

"Well, I do not know if I can afford it," he said. (That is something we hear a lot!)

"Well," I told him, "getting started with paperless is FREE. Do you think you can afford FREE?"

He just started laughing. "I think this is going to work out," he said.

All too often, dentists see improving their offices as a zero sum game—if they spend money here, they are going to have to cut back painfully somewhere else. This is not necessarily true—it is a fear-based feeling. The objective reality is that offices equipped with state-of-the-art technology attract and retain more patients.

They have a higher rate of treatment plan acceptance than those that look—and in fact are— out of date and out of touch.

A patient may not know exactly what each tool in your operatory does, but your patient sure can tell whether your office stacks up with others she has seen. Rather than focusing on what you need to subtract in order to gain, focus on the return on investment—your dividends will be extraordinary.

We handle the business side of things. That way the dentist can do clinical dentistry. Most dentists really do not want to deal with the business-related elements. They do not want to have to worry about bookkeeping, for example, and yet some of my dentists do their own. They stay in their offices until midnight, trying to figure the whole thing out, when they should really just hire a bookkeeper to come to the office and get things handled. There are plenty of bookkeepers who specialize in dental offices and understand the entire process. The bottom line is that dentists do not understand how much they can gain by modestly investing in their business. A lot of the problems that outmoded dental offices face cannot be handled as simply as bringing in a bookkeeper, however.

Dentists, by and large, would love to be able to walk into their offices in the morning, pull on their lab coats, and say, "Okay—who is my first patient?" without having to worry about the business side of dentistry. We automate the operatory, so that when the dentist sits down at the keyboard, the computer goes right to where he or she needs to go. When the X-ray is taken, the image goes right where it needs to go. Our dentists do not have to stress about making things work.

Not only do we see our clients improve the conveniences of the daily operations in their offices, but we also watch proudly as they become more profitable, and the investment pays for itself in a very short time frame. In one case, we put in dual monitors, and the doctor presented a case to a patient on those monitors for the first time. As a result, the patient really understood what was going on in his mouth, because he saw it up on the big screen that we had installed.

The doctor was able to close a $20,000 treatment plan, and the technology paid for itself immediately.

Or let's say you are installing a digital X-ray sensor for $5,000. Not only do you save $5,000 in consumables, but you are also getting rid of the headache that all those consumables represent. And so it goes throughout the office—the rule of thumb that I share with my clients is that technology often pays for itself in a matter of weeks, not months or years.

Some of our clients are building a brand-new office, so we work with them, and with their building contractors, from the start. In other cases, dentists upgrade their offices in phases. Either way, the technology makes an immediate and profound difference in the running of the office—and for the bottom line.

Typically, first we get the office's network up to speed and get the workstations running right, so your team members are not sitting on their elbows, waiting for an archaic computer to process information. Getting the network in, the servers up, the workstations in, the digital X-rays in … with each phase, you are going to see a tremendous change in how your office functions. By building a more stable technological foundation, it will be much easier to evolve with the times.

In the real world, keeping up with the Joneses is never a good idea. Our society, unfortunately, sometimes feels like it is running on an endless treadmill of materialism, where people are replacing perfectly good cars or tearing down perfectly good houses and building bigger ones just to impress the neighbors, who are busy with their own onslaught of new consumer items. Getting caught up in that materialistic cycle is nobody's idea of a good time. Your dental office is different, because patients can immediately tell the difference between an operatory that looks and feels state of the art and one that seems dated and out of synch with modern technology.

A patient can walk into an operatory that seems antiquated and unused. There is nothing going on in there, and yet that is where they are going to be treated?

That same patient will walk into another dentist's operatory with LEDs flashing on the computers and monitors.

The big screen will be up in place, and everything humming along nicely, and the client says, "Wow, this place has some technology built into it." And they feel more comfortable, and more secure, and they are more likely to trust the recommendation of the doctor when she presents a case. To put it simply, who do you think a patient would rather have working in his mouth, Dr. Betty Rubble ... or Dr. Buzz Lightyear? Who do you want to be?

We live in a technology-driven world. It is just that simple. Your patients are surrounded by technology all day long—in their workplaces and in their homes. Their children are masters of technology in ways that the average adult will never be.

Chances are excellent that the patients you desire the most have upgraded their personal computer, their home entertainment system, their cell phone or PDA, or some other critically important piece of technology within the last six months to a year.

How is a person like that expected to walk into an office that is clearly behind the times and agree to an expensive and complicated case?

Once I share that thought with doctors, suddenly they begin to realize that transforming their offices into state-of-the-art centers for the provision of top-flight dental care is not an option. It is a business necessity.

The lifeblood of a dental office is keeping your patients while attracting new ones—and above all, treatment plan acceptance. If you are seeking to sell your practice, one of the first questions you will be asked is how many new patients a month come through your door. If the response is that only about five or six new patients a month join the practice, that is pretty slow. We are talking about new people, people who have never been to your office before. A typical dental office might see 300 to 400 patients a month. Each one of those patients could refer one friend and business would double. A doctor who is only getting five or six new patients obviously is not generating much positive word of mouth.

By contrast, we just finished an office makeover for a dentist in Irvine, California, who sees on average sixty new patients a month.

What does his office have to offer? It's clean. It's up-to-date. It's bright and shiny. It has all of the latest, greatest technology in place to use for the benefit of the patients.

I mention all of this, because introducing new technology into your office doesn't just have an immediate payoff in terms of increasing your patient flow—and your cash flow.

It pays off once again when the time comes to sell your practice, because with the right technology in place, the referrals come quickly and easily.

Another important reason to consider updating technology in your office is that it gives you and your team members an opportunity to grow and learn. When people are not growing and learning they stagnate, and the office environment in which they operate becomes stagnant, too. Recently, we installed a new computer and a new digital X-ray system for one of our clients, and his chair side was giddy! She hadn't ever had a new toy to learn how to operate and work with. "This is going to look great on my resume!" she told us, and she named the particular products she was now using. "Wow, that's great!"

What did her resume look like before that? Plain Jane. If she's got all the latest toys to play with, do you think she's going to be updating her resume? So we see that another important benefit of bringing in new technology is that you retain your staff members at a greater rate, because they are more enthusiastic about coming into the office. And that sense of enthusiasm spills over into your patient base as well.

We install and integrate technology; we also provide consulting services for dentists to help ensure that as they add new technology, whether from us or from someone else, they and their teams know exactly how to operate and get the most from it.

We also have the ability to manage our doctors' systems remotely. This means that if a computer glitch suddenly arises in your system, you call us.

We can get inside your system from our office, identify the glitch, and repair it immediately, instead of having your whole office losing days or even weeks until the problem is identified and repaired. That aspect of our service alone separates us from our competitors and makes us incredibly valuable to our clients.

So whether you are a dentist at the beginning of your career, looking to make maximum impact with the best possible office, or you are looking to upgrade your office in mid-career, or even position your practice for sale to an associate or another dentist, we can help.

I have never heard any of our clients come back to us and say that the money they invested in technology didn't come back to them immediately—and many times over. I understand that you are taking a leap when you upgrade, and that you are moving away from "the way we've always done it around here."

I want to put the idea in your mind that dentistry can be even more enjoyable, service-oriented, and lucrative—for you and for your team—when you've got the right technology in place. You will offer confidence to your patients and your team that everything is happening the way it is supposed to happen, when it is supposed to happen.

To put it simply, do you want to be perceived as Dr. Betty Rubble or as Dr. Buzz Lightyear? Your patients are waiting for you to take them out of Bedrock ... and to the future ... and beyond!

Chapter 2
The Office Your Patients Expect You to Have

"The appearance of your office indicates the type and quality of the treatment you provide."— James Rotondo

The key to gaining referrals and also treatment plan acceptance from your current patients does not solely rest on how good you are as a practitioner. It is also largely about how comfortable and confident your office makes your patients feel.

The main goal is to create an office that is warm and inviting, an office that makes you feel welcome. Ideally, the environment is light and airy, not dark, drab and institutionalized. I visited an office a little while ago that has enormous plush chairs and healthy green plants. It was calming, yet safe and happy. I felt right at home.

It is a delicate balancing act though, since a lot of patients do not necessarily understand that a dentist runs a **business**. Normally, a patient sees their doctor because they have a problem, not because the doctor needs to make money. And the same thing happens with a dentist. If you actually pointed out to a patient that the dentist is trying to run a business, the patient would likely say, "You are right! I never thought about it!"

So you never want your lobby to feel as if you are there to take the patient's money. When Fred and Wilma walk into a dental office, they want to feel comfortable, not pressured to fork out their money.

They are there because they've got a problem. They've got a cavity, and they are coming to you so you can fill it. They do not realize that it is your business to fill it, and you are going to make money doing it, and that is how you make your living. I know that might sound obvious, but it is very true. They come to you to solve a problem. They may not be qualified to judge the quality of your dental work. But they sure know how they feel when they are visiting your office.

A patient's senses are of utmost importance when they first walk into the reception area. It is important, then, to cater to their senses at the onset of their experience with you. It is all about what they feel when they first walk in the door. Does your office look like an accommodating and warm place? Does it look inviting? Does it look friendly? In an ideal world, patients walk into the reception room and think, "Wow. This place is really nice. I can hang out here awhile." They are not going to tell *you* that, but that is what is going through their minds.

If you've got a vinyl floor and white walls, your office does not reflect that you do high-end cosmetic dentistry.

Your office has to reflect the work that you do and the patient needs to see it. Patients gain confidence visually and aesthetically. Modern and innovative offices reflect your abilities and personality. What does *your* office suggest about your abilities?

Let us begin by talking about your reception area. You can enhance this space by installing a television, getting new furniture, or even changing the lights.

Brighten the whole place; use different colored light bulbs to color correct the room so that it feels much more pleasing. Show your patients that you care. If they feel like you care about their comfort while they wait, they will have confidence in your ability to care for them once they are in your chair.

After the initial visual impression that the atmosphere in your reception area creates, the focus shifts to the other senses. Does it smell like a dental office? Nobody wants that! What are the sounds the patients hear? Do they hear the whining and whirling of handpieces, conversations, the obnoxious air conditioner going full blast, or do they hear light and relaxing music? It is important to make the patients feel like they are the only ones there. A nice, calm, and easygoing reception room gives your patients that exclusive feeling.

Inevitably, in terms of sound, some office spaces are easier to renovate than others. Some are larger and have thicker walls, which are better for soundproofing.

When you build your office, you have to actually plan for sound muting. As an example, when a pediatric office in Irvine was installing drywall, we planned ahead and used soundproof insulation between the walls. When the drywall was installed, we hung sound-muting board on the wall. Essentially, it was a sandwich of materials to deaden the noise. You could speak loudly and nobody in the office would hear you. And because the noises are not heard, it creates that ambiance that is so desired. Calm, soothing, relaxing, and inviting. Tranquil, if you will.

The same goes for sound in the reception room. I always suggest ceiling insulation, insulation around the air fittings, wall insulation, and door insulation. I always seek to find a way to make the area a little more quiet. Maybe a nice big throw rug will make a difference. Patients do not want to listen to someone else receiving treatment while they wait to receive their own. Remember, the objective is tranquil, calm, and comfortable. And yes, it is going to be kind of difficult to do, but you have to think about the materials that make up the office that will make it the way you want it to be.

Now let us go chairside and talk about the tools you use. By tools, I refer to your delivery systems and handpieces. You might be thinking that you have the same tools as all of the other dentists, so what is the difference? You are right—dentists are equal in the fact that they all have the same basic toolset. I have found, however, that the quality of a dentist's tools, and his ability to correctly use those tools, correlates to the quality of his work. The opposite is true, too. This holds true for many other services and trades in the world; the better your equipment, the better your results will be. If you are using your feet to operate your tools, that is a great indication that it is time to upgrade.

I know that you are asking, "What's the big deal?" The tools are all able to blow air. They all have water with which to rinse the patient's mouth. They all have suction. And all dentists have chairs, handpieces, and X-ray machines.

But in the dentistry business (yes, your practice is a business, remember?), it is not enough to be merely equal with your competitors. You have to excel.

You have to stand out in order to attract new patients. You have to be unique.

The caliber of your tools is what your patient observes and experiences. It is how you design your operatory that makes your business unique.

When patients enter your office, will they see all the instruments of "pain" that you are going to use on them ... all spread out on the counter ready for you to use? Or will they be afforded the opportunity to sit down in a comfortable chair, with no painful tools in sight, because they are stored in the aesthetically pleasing cabinets? No hose, no obtrusive lights. Everything is calm and tranquil. Which invites more confidence and comfort? Which would you prefer, if you were a patient?

Comfort and confidence are hard things to put a price on. When you visit a really nice office, you feel like you are stepping into a plush expensive car rather than a budget model. And it makes you feel a little happier to think that you are being treated as well as the place looks.

Equal or unique? Which do you want to be? There are dentists who accept the idea that patients will come and patients will go, and they are comfortable with that.

There are other dentists who like the idea of having patients stay with them for years and years, because of the friendship and rapport, quality of service, comfort and ease, and confidence the patients have that they are well taken care of. Your willingness to design an inviting environment, in order to make the patient feel comfortable, will set you apart.

Some dentists with whom we have worked, actually have chairs with built-in massage functions. Some have heat. Obviously, those are nice luxuries that are not necessary, but they are options and they do convey a poignant message. When you apply the term "spa," you think about going to get a facial and massage, relaxing to nice music and listening to a serene water fountain. More and more of our high-end dental offices are becoming dental spas. There are medical spas, and now there are dental spas. You can get your teeth worked on while you are getting a manicure. That is a neat thing.

There are all kinds of things that dentists can do to enhance the patient's experience. Digital X-ray machines make the work easier, but they also show patients that you are technologically advanced.

The chair quality, the lighting, the music, the decorations, the environment, and the little extra things all make a difference. I have worked with doctors who have really taken it to the next level. They've told me, "We want aromatherapy units hidden throughout the office so we can make sure the patients are as calm and comfortable as possible." Add a massage chair to the aromatherapy and who would not want to come back? That sounds much nicer than a dark, dingy operatory with plastic-covered chairs, loud noises, and tools on the counter.

One of our clients took the entire process to a new level by traveling around to a large number of cities throughout the world, and photographing the lobbies of the nicest hotels he could find. With the pictures in hand, he hired an interior designer to combine the ideas for him and create a very inviting environment that would be considered five-star. It worked. WOW, what an office. And NO, it did not cost millions of dollars.

Now let us talk about the importance of technology.

More and more dental chairs have televisions or some type of audio system on them. Maybe even a wireless headset.

I have one dentist who opted for goggles that allow the patient to view a 50-inch plasma screen—dentistry and movies all in one. Technology is a selling point, especially if the patient has to wait in the dental chair a few minutes to see you. If you have a television, I suggest you hand the remote to the patient so he can browse the stations. This is just one more thing to make patients feel comfortable and at home.

Some dental offices run a closed-circuit cable television loop. They might have one channel that runs a loop for a kids' station, another channel for adults to watch, and another that runs patient education videos.

These look like you are watching an interview on TV, but it is really patient education regarding treatment procedures and options. People watch and learn about how root canals help teeth, and are interested in exploring it further. Young adults and children are accustomed to a constant feed of information via technology such as Internet and TV. They will be more comfortable, and so will their parents, in an office that accommodates their lifestyle. Adopting the latest technology with regard to your chair is essential.

Technology is neat. Patients love it. When a patient's lying there, watching TV and relaxing, and then you offer to show an X-ray, it is great to have the capability to simply slide it up onto that TV with a flip of the remote. Patients enjoy that kind of thing and respect you for it. I once interviewed a patient who said, "Wow. I was just watching TV and sitting in the chair, and then on the same screen the dentist showed me my X-ray. I was able to see what he needed to show me. And I felt much more educated about the treatment he was prescribing."

Digital is one way to make those X-rays easily visible for your patient. Intraoral cameras are another imaging option, which allows dentists to put a camera in the patient's mouth to take a picture. They can then view it on their screen; look at it for a second; change the colors, contrast, and brightness; and even crop it a little, if they wish. Or they can send it to the television and show it to the patient. Patients feel like they are getting advanced technological treatment, and they are.

The entertainment is an added bonus. Meanwhile, the doctor is utilizing those services to actually sell treatment plans.

All of this together makes for a productive, impressive technological environment.

"Treatment plan acceptance has certainly changed for the better in [the] days since we have installed the monitors for the patients to see. I have been able to [obtain] acceptance on more cases, and even more difficult cases to explain. The patient monitor is worth a million words—try to explain a crack in a molar versus showing the crack in the molar. The patient has nothing to say but yes—let's get it fixed."

—JV, Southern California

TV dictates to a very high degree your patients' expectations about what dental offices should look and feel like. Patients are learning a lot from TV! When they watch sitcoms and dramas, they see what an up-to-date office can look like. People see a commercial about teeth whitening products, and which system works the best, and they are learning about what to ask their dentists.

The Wellness Hour is a cable TV show frequently featuring dentists. On one episode, the doctor talked about using implant technology for denture replacement, so that dentures do not fall out or need adhesives. The ads and marketing are prevalent. They are in printed magazines and on Internet sites. I mention this because if you know what people expect, you have a better chance of obtaining their business. If you have what they expect, you can market yourself. Use the best and latest technology and the best practice methods, and you are in an excellent position for a successful business.

We've talked about the feeling your office creates and the expectations your patients bring to the experience of dentistry today. Now let us talk about another critically important subject—patient information privacy.

With the extensive amount of personal information stored via technology, it is imperative to make sure it is kept safe. Patients make an assumption about safety based on the quality of the office. They often assume that if the office is organized, their information is secure.

That is not enough! It is important for you to guarantee that their information is safe.

One thing that I like to see a dentist's office do is release a little press release: "We upgraded the security of your identity, and these are the things that we did in order to do that.

In an effort to protect you and to work in line with HIPAA compliancy, we want you to rest assured that your information is privileged and safe."

Going paperless is ideal. It is fantastic for a couple of reasons. The initial reason to go paperless is to stop spending money on consumable products. You will not need to buy paper as much as you did. You will not need charting folders, rubber stamps, labels, and whatever else you've bought in the past. You will immediately save money. Additionally, going paperless helps save the environment. You also need to tell your patients that by utilizing the newest technology available, your office is going to better serve them. They need to know that their information will be backed up and safe. You cannot back up a paper chart, but you can back up a server.

A lot of the dentists are terrified to go paperless, and I understand their concerns. We'll discuss the question of going paperless in Chapter 11.

If we were making a video about organizing your charts, I'd have a little, slightly overweight doctor in a lab coat, wearing glasses that have tape in the middle of the frame. He would push his glasses up while dropping files, as he is coming in to talk to you about your procedure.

It is unprofessional for a doctor to approach a patient carrying a chart five or six inches thick, because it makes the patient seem as though he has a lot of problems.

True, the patient might have bad teeth, but those dentists have a bad filing system! If a dentist cannot keep his charts in order, it destroys the patient's confidence that he can work effectively on his teeth. It can be really irritating for patients when a doctor flips through the chart to figure out what he needs to discuss and do. With technology, however, a dentist has the information readily accessible. Information technology is well worth the investment, for this reason alone.

Charting has to be done in a manner that is defensible in court. Let us say you use a piece of software with the option of a paperless signature tablet, just as you would use with the credit card at the grocery store.

It allows you to show your patients the video and then have them sign the signature tablet for the informed consent for treatment. With some software packages you have the ability to manipulate the signature; you can cut it, copy it, crop it, resize it, and even paste it on another form if you so choose.

Unfortunately, this is not defensible in court because it can be easily copied or reproduced without your authorization. Patterson EagleSoft is just one of the many Practice Management packages that capture and encrypt the signature so that it cannot be altered in any way. I hope you will agree with me that high-end technology is well worth the investment, to protect the patient's confidence in you and to protect your own legal position.

Safety cameras and other surveillance equipment are other options that you have. Some dentists have them and some do not. A lot of dentists think that it is going overboard to install such equipment, but there are those who want the video surveillance.

They want to cover their practice and keep things safe. They want to make sure that patients do not take advantage and claim accidents that didn't happen. They also want to make sure that people in the office do not do things they should not do. They want to watch the transaction counters and the reception area or lobby. They want to know what is going on. This is entirely for you to decide. If you choose to have cameras installed, remember to put a plaque up that tells people that video surveillance is taking place. A lot of dentists do not do that, but they've got cameras in the ceiling. That may open them up to some legal exposure.

Today's dental patients have all kinds of expectations when they come to you. They expect to be safe, they expect innovative technology, they expect hygienic care, but, most of all, they expect you to Care!

There are a lot of dentists out there, trust me, who do not care and it shows. They just really don't. If they can get an instrument in a patient's mouth, that means that they are charging the insurance company. That is all they care about.

That is not you. You want to provide the best care in the most soothing, up-to-date environment. From the look of the reception area or lobby to the sound of the office, from the technology that inspires confidence in you to the dental chair that offers massage and TV, and from the information technology that puts you in command of your information instead of at the mercy of stacks of unruly charts, the patient wants you to have the best … so that he can be sure that he is getting the best care. And that is when he'll be most receptive to accept your case … and pay you what you are truly worth.

Chapter 3

Five Technology Changes You Can Make Right Now

The dentists I meet would love to put new technology into their offices right away, because they understand that new technology translates into new patients, happier patients, and increased case conversions. The only thing the dentists do not want to do is spend a lot of money.

The good news is that they don't have to.

In this chapter, I want to share with you five technology changes and upgrades you can make right away that will have a dramatic and immediate impact on your bottom line, not to mention on the morale of your team members and the attitude of your patients to the treatment you present.

The modern dental 'office contains a virtual catalog of technology components, each of which impacts day-to-day efficiency and productivity, and each of which serves a specific function. Before we address the five technology changes you can make immediately, I'd like to first detail the different features—technological and otherwise—of the modern dental 'office, so that you can understand how each impacts the workplace.

Let us start with the reception area, or the lobby, the first room that patients experience. Almost all lobbies have a large-screen television, for a variety of reasons. Some use televisions to entertain patients while they wait, usually with HGTV, headline news, or a movie from a pre-purchased library.

Tranquil scenery—waterfalls, ocean waves, idyllic destinations—are also commonly played on the television, offering background sounds that both soothe and also mask the distracting sounds of real life.

Other offices prefer to be more proactive and opt to showcase patient education software—looping, long-running production that resembles a television show.

The purpose is to introduce certain aspects of dentistry—veneers, dental implants, etc. Think of it as an entertaining infomercial for the dental industry.

In addition to the television, many lobbies now have wireless Internet access, as a convenience for patients. Whether they are waiting for their own treatment or that of their spouse or children, visitors are afforded the opportunity to pass time on their laptop. After logging in with the office password, displayed on a professionally printed sign, people can use the Internet to work while they wait. The simple gesture of offering Wi-Fi can paint your practice as generous and considerate in your patients' eyes.

But even beyond entertaining, there are ways to make an impression before your patients even start to experience the quality of your service.

Several manufacturers now offer software that allows patients to check in without needing to wait for someone at reception.

The current leaders in this field, Dentrix, Patterson EagleSoft and Dolphin Management, allow the interaction to take place either via kiosk-style computers or tablet PCs.

They can even prompt the patient to provide updated health history records through an on-screen form.

Not only does this enhance efficiency, but it also provides better accountability for the maintenance of patient records.

The check-in software also allows the use of signature tablets—like those found on supermarket credit card machines or UPS confirmation clipboards—or even fingerprint readers, as a means to best accommodate clients. Built into the front desk it is not only efficient but also pretty darn cool, and the patients love it too.

Once the patient has checked in, other features come into play, namely the top-notch sound system or the aforementioned flat screen television. The patient may also notice a feature that is becoming increasingly popular in the medical field: the self-service bar and refreshment center. Sort of the equivalent of a hotel mini-bar—without the alcohol or outrageous surcharges—the refreshment bar offers light snacks, coffee, tea, juice, and bottled water.

Some of the items are even packaged with the logo of the medical practice, with the hope that the products will be taken outside the office to increase the marketing exposure. Some doctors even go beyond the branded bottled water to offer fresh-baked cookies. Sodas may be verboten, but Otis Spunkmeyer is becoming an increasingly common sight in dental offices. Ahh, the smell of chocolate chip cookies fresh out of the oven. A self-service refreshment bar may not incorporate space-age technology, but it does showcase a forward-thinking mindset of catering to the patient and making the doctor's office a more pleasant place to visit—a nominal expense that yields immeasurable payback.

When the patient is called into the office, he or she will most likely see the receptionist and the receptionist's computer. If any of the equipment looks outdated, with a hulking tube monitor cluttering the desk instead of a sleek flat-panel screen, the patient will most assuredly form a negative opinion of the office's systems.

Clunky printers, fax machines, and other prehistoric-looking equipment can lead to similar patient disapproval, and also cause them to wonder if your medical equipment is equally antiquated. Any of the equipment that is readily visible to the patient should be as clean and up-to-date as possible. Also let's not forget that the person at the front desk needs to be highly efficient and proficient with the use of the computer, software, and all other necessary technology. Training Training Training ...

Some doctors prefer cutting-edge equipment—and they make certain the patient knows it. Monitor-mounted cameras are becoming de rigueur in the modern medical office, not just for keeping up appearances, but also for practical purposes.

The same cameras that teens use to video chat with their friends are given a more pragmatic application in the medical office, where they are used to snap photos of patients to add to their files. Facilitating patient recognition, photos provide a much higher level of customer service and interaction, which in turn leads to a more satisfied feeling of connection on the part of the patient.

For the dentist, it adds an extra layer of security, ensuring that the chart he or she is reading corresponds to the patient seated in the chair.

After the lobby, the consultation office stands to make an impression on patients, especially first time patients. The consultation room is similar to a private office where an office manager or accounts manager—not usually the dentist himself—discusses the treatment the doctor has planned. After the treatment coordinator (as the person in this role is often called) has finished the explanation, the doctor, if needed, is summoned to answer any final or advanced questions.

A number of doctors view the consultation room as a place to perform the hard sell, which explains the strategic placement of its innovative and extravagant equipment.

Gleaming new printers, scanners, cameras, and signature tablets provide expedience in documentation, should the patient agree to the treatment. In the consultation room, payments can be made, schedules printed, and pictures taken—everything that can be done at reception.

The objective is to keep the patient in the room until all necessary documentation is complete.

I am a huge proponent of utilizing tools that help demonstrate the prescribed treatment plan. Dual-monitor systems, yet another innovative feature in the consultation room, function to display the patient's chart on one screen and X-rays on the other. It is almost as if the consultation room were half front desk, half operatory.

Contrary to what you might think, the doctor's private office doesn't boast the high-tech gadgetry found throughout the rest of the office. Of course it has the essentials—computer, printer, fax machine—but aside from a higher-powered computer, that is about it. Some doctors choose to use the consultation room as their office, and vice versa, in order to make the maximum use of space. In such cases, the same rules apply as those for the regular consultation room.

However, although a patient will rarely see a doctor's office, that does not mean you should neglect this room.

The doctor, too, needs a place of respite, a sanctuary during lunch hour, or even while performing regular business tasks such as billing or reviewing charts. What's more, the doctor needs a place to entertain colleagues. You do not want to shortchange yourself with a too-small office that cannot accommodate a few business associates for meetings, or one that is so spartan you never feel completely at ease. We can help you to strike the balance between austere and over-the-top.

Next step: the operatory, where chairside charting has become the norm. I cannot stress how important it is to have a chairside computer. It is a multi-functional piece that demonstrates progressiveness and enhances efficiency.

Digital X-rays are one of the chairside computer's most important functions. Patients who are even remotely familiar with current medical practices know that film X-rays subject patients to 50 percent more radiation than their digital counterparts. Such exposure is completely unnecessary. Digital X-rays are a necessity; thus, the chairside computer is necessary. It facilitates the image capture and is the main connection point for the digital X-ray sensor.

I have personally been in an office and watched a "new" patient get out of the chair and leave based solely on the use of analog and not digital X-rays.

An intraoral camera is another key component of the chairside computer setup. Rather than taking an X-ray, the dentist can use the intraoral camera to take an up-close photo of a broken tooth to show the patient. If they choose, patients can watch a screen to see the doctor at work. While the doctor and patient view the same image, the information surrounding the image is usually quite different, and the doctor can make available additional information as he sees fit. With the problem area highlighted on the screen, the doctor can discuss treatment options and help the patient decide on a path for treatment.

The second monitor, the one the patient views, also serves as a TV screen. If a patient has to wait on the doctor—or even if the procedure itself, such as a Zoom treatment, requires additional time—the television is accessible. As a distracter during treatment that may be unpleasant, the television invites comfort and relaxation.

And because the patient monitor can display television, it can also display patient education videos. As evidenced, strategically placed TV screens are multipurpose and multifunctional. They save the doctor time, they pique patient interest, they enhance sales, they entertain and educate, and, because they educate, they alleviate patient apprehension.

The operatory is designed to be the place of treatment, as well as a pseudo-consultation room where dentists can close sales—a process dentists refer to as "treatment plan acceptance." If all goes well, the dentist will get the patient's acceptance while she is still seated in the chair. Savvy doctors might even try to motivate the patient to have the procedure done immediately. "The procedure only takes twenty minutes," says the sales-minded dentist, "and you are already here. If you have another twenty minutes, we can get it over with right now. No need for a return visit."

Because that is what a dentist wants to do. He wants to get you in, treat you, get the treatment plan acceptance, and move forward.

That is an excellent sales technique. In the event of a more complex (and expensive) case, however—like full mouth reconstruction, implants, veneers, or orthodontics—it makes sense to bring the patient into a consultation room and discuss the matter in depth there. A patient will rarely accept a complex treatment plan while sitting (or lying down) in your operatory. Sitting upright in a chair versus being in a vulnerable reclined position allows the patient to feel that there is mutual respect in the decision-making process. Additionally, in large treatment plans, touchy financial discussions may need to take place.

In addition to the operatory, X-ray booths are becoming increasingly popular. Using an X-ray booth may seem to be old school but is proving to be a time-saver.

The booth eliminates that waste of time. An upright dental chair with a headrest is installed in a room slightly smaller than a regular operatory, where computer and digital X-ray equipment are set up.

Rather than wasting time in an actual dental chair, patients are whisked to the X-ray room, then back to the lobby to await the results. When an operatory becomes available, the patient is invited to return. The smoothness this creates enables the doctor to clock more treatment minutes per dental chair, rather than X-ray minutes. This also allows for the doctor to sit in the comfort of his or her office to quickly review the X-rays.

In the more up-to-date offices, the X-ray booths include intraoral cameras as well as Pan/Ceph, or Panoramic Cephalometric X-ray machines, so that the dentist can produce an image of all the patient's teeth, as well as the nasal area, sinuses, jaw joints, and surrounding bone—with much less radiation. For those who wish to step even higher, more cutting-edge doctors are installing 3-D, i-CAT style X-ray units, a bit more money but the benefits far outweigh the cost.

X-ray booths equip the dentist with the option of offering high-end digital camera work, which may include "smile photographs," photographs of your teeth as a whole set to demonstrate your bite.

The patient's experience in the X-ray booth is that of a highly efficient dental office, one that allows for a whole barrage of diagnostics in one sitting, and without the patient having to wait in the operatory chair.

"Utilizing the X-ray booth instead of an operatory chair, I am able to review the patients X-rays while the patient is getting a cleaning. I can examine the X-rays from the comfort of my private office, or anywhere for that matter, and therefore I am far more informed when I approach the patient. I have more time to develop my ideas on treatment if treatment is needed—no more snap decisions based on a quick look, while the patient waits."—RH, Southern California

Technology is great and undoubtedly enhances patient experiences. But it can only do so much; your staff needs to be happy, too. I have seen a trend in which doctors' offices are raising the expectations of their staff—but staffs are also expecting more from their boss and workplace. While doctors cite computer literacy as one of the top skills expected of their office staff, employees now expect their workplace to provide them with the minor conveniences of their homes. Hence, the staff lounge.

In any workplace that entails a large amount of client interaction, the staff need a place of refuge, somewhere to rest that is out of patient sight. Staff members need to eat meals, make private phone calls, and get a few moments of hard-earned rest and relaxation. Most every one of the new offices we are building has allowed for a well-equipped staff lounge, whether it be a top-of-the-line break room—outfitted with every cooking gadget from microwaves to sub-zero refrigerators—or simply a counter and barstools for lunchtime. But the trend seems to hint that the more the office expects of their employees, the more it is willing to give in return.

Some staff lounges have Wi-Fi and computer stations separate from the office network, solely for personal use. Some have state-of-the-art sound systems, or even the same well-stocked self-service bars offered to the patients in the lobby. I have even seen practices that go so far as to have regular employee barbecues, complete with rib eye steak and fresh corn on the cob.

To some practices this may sound like a huge financial outlay, but I can assure you that when employees are happy, they are far more loyal. And a happy staff is as evident to the boss as it is to the patients. It is something you cannot put a price tag on.

"We spend more time together and awake than we spend with our families, why shouldn't we have fun together as a family does. A family that eats together stays together."—WD, Southern California

So technology and similar advancements really affect three different groups of people: the patients, the doctors, and the staff. When you look at it that way, how can you afford *not* to upgrade?

And that brings us to the crux of this chapter: the five technology changes you can make *right now*.

1.   Let's start with the **dual-monitor system**, which was described as a vital component of an efficient operatory and even the consultation room. A dual-monitor system is an inexpensive way to increase your sales, because it allows for faster and more frequent acceptance of treatment plans.

A single screen just will not cut it, because it fails to accommodate the patient and forces him or her to move in order to view the doctor's monitor.

Rather than adding to the inconvenience and discomfort of the patient, a second monitor can be attached to the dental chair. In the case of chairs not equipped to handle a monitor, a properly-sized wall monitor is a more than acceptable—and far less expensive—option. With the addition of the second monitor, the patient can watch television, and the dentist can present digital X-rays and treatment plans in a much more effective way. For about $2,000 per operatory—barely more than the cost of a filling— you can install a dual-monitor system into an operatory. With the increase in treatment plan acceptance, the whole system could pay for itself in less than a day.

2.   The next item on your list should be upgrading or adding computers. Patients and staff do not like to wait on slow computers. You might as well plead that the dog ate your schedule book, because it is an equally poor defense. Upgrading your office computers will impress your patients and optimize staff time.

If you lost ten minutes on every patient over the course of the day, at the end of the month you'd have lost a few hours. In the course of a year, that can translate to a full week of lost time—all because your computers are too slow.

A computer upgrade often does not involve much more than installing more memory or changing the network or video card. For newer computers, one or more of these three upgrades can save the day. However, in older systems this might not be an option. If a computer is more than three years old, get a new one. Old ones are unacceptable, and are prone to technological Alzheimer's.

In the long run, a complete upgrade of the entire computer will cost you far less than what your office will be losing in terms of time—and reputation.

3.   Digital X-ray sensors are a must. The cost can widely vary—from as little as $5,000 per sensor, depending on the quality and your own personal deal—but I cannot emphasize how important this investment will be to your practice. Start off with one set and move it from operatory to operatory, as needed. You will not be disappointed.

No matter how many sets you buy off the bat, you will need to have your operatories prepared to use digital X-ray sensors. This generally involves installing the proper cables and computer preparations, which usually costs about $1,000 per area, whether that be an operatory proper or X-ray booth.

4.   As with the digital X-ray sensors, digital intraoral cameras require some degree of cabling—the exact same cabling for each, in fact. If your operatory has already been cabled for X-rays, then by default you are already wired for intraoral cameras, which cost anywhere from $1,000 to $6,000.

But the investment in an intraoral camera goes back to case acceptance. When a patient truly understands his or her particular dental dilemma, he or she is more likely to agree to the solution—which often can be shown with the aid of an intraoral camera. "So that is what that sharp spot is in my mouth!" says the patient, seeing the pointy part of a broken tooth for the first time. "Let's fix it!"

5.   The last item on the list is the case-presentation software. There are several brands that, with just a few keystrokes, enable the dentist to build a customized presentation that explains to the patient his or her particular problem and how the dentist proposes to treat it. Some doctors, in an attempt to avoid purchasing additional software, will futz with compiling the patient's digital images into a PowerPoint presentation.

While I applaud their ingenuity, it simply does not make sense to waste that amount of time on a process that can be far more easily replicated with software built expressly for that purpose.

With case-presentation software, a dentist need only answer a few simple questions on the monitor, then wait for the presentation to compile. If a 35-year-old male patient needs an implant on tooth #7, a doctor can enter his information and in just a few moments have a fully animated presentation of the required procedure for the patient's viewing pleasure. The cost of this type of software can vary from $1,000 to $5,000 depending on the complexity.

Perhaps in the next edition of this book, I will have additional information on a new practice I have only just recently seen. Since it is so new, I have no way of knowing yet whether or not it actually works. But I think it is worth mentioning.

One of my clients recently decided to transform each of his operatories into a stand-alone, full-service desk. For example, if a patient just finished getting a filling, the doctor could schedule an appointment, print out an appointment reminder, and accept payment for the services—all while the patient is still feeling groggy in the chair. The doctor hopes not only to improve the patient experience but also to cut office headcount.

I am not sure yet if this system will work, but the idea intrigues me. Rest assured that if it is successful, you will be hearing about it from me.

You now have the tools to make your own decision about how to upgrade your office. You may have always wanted to upgrade but hesitated because you feared you'd spend money in the wrong places or were afraid of being sold on something you didn't really need. But now you have the knowledge to bring your practice up to speed and to choose the tools that will put more money in your pocket *right now*. You can be confident that you can go out and do this, both for your own reputation and that of your business. And if you still have questions, I am just a phone call away.

Chapter 4

It's Easier Than You Might Think!

Trust me: You do not need an Ivy League education to be the top dentist in town. Your office equipment says much more about your practice than any framed degree ever could. Upgrading equipment may not always come cheaply, but the return on investment can be enormous—if you make the right choices.

Adding technology to your office enables you to learn a new treatment or process that will enhance your abilities to make higher profits. It is kind of like being a mechanic. You may know how to swap out an engine, but if you do not have a lift to raise the car, you cannot perform the service. Having the lift allows the mechanic to provide numerous additional services that bring in much more money than the equipment cost to begin with.

I visited a doctor recently—I will call him Dr. Fogey—who didn't want to upgrade to digital X-rays or any other forward-thinking practices. In a polite manner, I asked him how old he was, and Dr. Fogey replied that he was pushing 65. "That is great," I said. "Are you going to transition out and retire?" The doctor replied that he was thinking of picking up an associate somewhere down the line. That is when I broke the news to him. "That is a wonderful goal to strive for, but the current state of your office is not going to attract top-quality associates." Dr. Fogey went on to explain that he did not want to, nor did he feel he could learn all the procedures the new equipment would require. I asked him why he had hired me in the first place, and it turns out he just wanted a simple server and workstation installed in the back office.

I didn't push the matter, even though I knew that Dr. Fogey's reluctance to upgrade would keep his business from growing, and might even cause him to lose the patients he already had. Without the proper equipment, Dr. Fogey will be unable to offer the same new treatments as his competitors, and his patients might just decide to use a dentist who has not frozen his practice in 1995. He probably also will not get the pick of the litter when it comes to assistants, since new graduates are trained on the newest technology and expect to have that equipment available at their office.

It is not just that Dr. Fogey is missing out on the opportunity to enhance his appearance. His patients are missing out on the opportunity to see what he sees when he is working on them. Even the least technologically-equipped dentist can look in your mouth, see a problem, and decide on a treatment. But trying to describe what you are seeing to a patient is a completely different story. Without seeing what you see, the patient must go on blind trust, as we discussed in Chapter 1.

Just down the road is a slightly younger doctor—whom I will call Dr. Modern—who has a technologically up-to-date office and, not so coincidentally, a young associate who is thrilled to be working with all the latest equipment—digital X-rays, intraoral cameras, the works. Dr. Modern and I spoke about upgrading his existing intraoral cameras to ones that would allow him to do a live feed on the patient's monitor and then freeze-frame the image to store on a computer. Who do you think would win the patient's trust and understanding, Dr. Fogey or Dr. Modern?

It is human nature to harp on a negative experience more than we'd praise a positive one, so the amount of damage that can be done by even one dissatisfied patient can be exponential. People talk with their friends about dentists well beyond just offering referrals, especially if they have just seen a new piece of technology or undergone an extensive procedure. Women in particular discuss their dentists, especially if they have just had a cosmetic treatment or a cleaning that made their teeth look especially good. If your office is so far behind the times that your equipment might as well be a hammer and chisel, you are in danger of having negative word of mouth spread to your potential client base. You simply cannot afford that smear on your reputation. Patients can't tell a good composite filling from a mediocre one. But they can tell a cutting-edge office from one that is behind the times.

Your goal is to be the doctor recommended by patients who have tried your newly added treatments. Staying at the head of the game means that you just might be the only doctor in the neighborhood offering a certain treatment, so even if you are not mentioned by name, patients will find you. Some of the more popular new treatments include upgraded veneers, better restorations, and dental implants, including both teeth and dentures— none of which are particularly difficult but which provide additional options to patients without their having to see a specialist.

Let's say Dr. Fogey decides to upgrade his office so that he now has computers in the front and back, including chairside stations and digital X-rays. If the doctor then decided to take a three-day hands-on class on dental implants, he is now equipped to take a digital X-ray that electronically measures where the implant will go, which he can then show to his patient. A doctor without digital radiography would be far more hesitant to perform such a procedure, since X-rays must be taken each step of the way. Implant cases are not particularly difficult, but without the proper equipment they can be unnecessarily long, since you have to wait each time you take an analog film X-ray. Imagine the view if you have a 3-D system; many more treatment options become available.

True, there are doctors who perform implant procedures the old-school way, but if a patient knew how much easier on them it would be with the latest equipment, he would not hesitate to hightail it to another office. It is not just money that is at stake, but a patient's comfort and health. Given how fearful some patients are of the dentist, you should try to assuage their apprehension by offering the most comfortable treatment available. Imagine if your own dentist said, "I am not going to bother learning that new, no-pain cavity-filling process. I prefer a challenge!" Not very reassuring, is it?

Of course, with today's technology being as complex as it is, some dentists—especially older ones—might harbor their own fears. If they cannot even figure out how to work their television remote, the thought of a whole office of new technology can be rather daunting. But believe it or not, dental technology is often far less complicated than placing a call on your cell phone, with most pieces of equipment requiring only a few mouse clicks. We would never expect a dentist to be a computer whiz—that is what *we* are here for.

Let me give you an example of just how easy the process can be. Say you want to take an X-ray. You simply properly place the digital sensor, align the head *(be sure to lower the exposure time),* and hit the button on the wall. Voilà! The image appears right on the screen. I do not think we could make it any easier than a two-step process.

Think of it as like buying a new car. It is not that your old vehicle was any easier to drive—in some cases, it might be just the opposite—but you do have to get used to where all the controls are, so that you do not turn on your windshield wipers when you go to make a left turn. Not only does a new car come with features to make it more efficient, such as GPS or a rearview camera, but it is also much safer than your previous ride. The same holds true for dental equipment.

To continue the analogy, the new car might even be more cost-efficient, getting you more miles per gallon. With new dental equipment, you can still charge the patient the same amount per treatment, but you are now performing the procedure in much less time and with less expense. By keeping up with technology, you can actually make your practice more profitable.

Let's use dental implants as an example. Many doctors who haven't upgraded their equipment simply will not do implants, but rather will refer their patients to a specialist after they have already paid for a consultation and X-rays. The specialist will then charge for another set of X-rays—and douse the patient with a second round of radiation—before performing the procedure. All in all, an implant with a crown could run between $3,000 and $5,000.

In no way am I saying that the specialist is not necessary, but the trend seems to be with proper case selection the easier implants are being performed by the general dentist. I would simply like to see that the general dentist has the proper technology equipment to take on such a challenge.

Dr. Modern is equipped with the proper technology and so can perform that same procedure in his office in less than half an hour for each of two visits: one for the initial implant and one a few months later to install the crown. For forty minutes of work, he grosses roughly $4,000.

Dr. Fogey, on the other hand, is not going to offer an implant, but rather offers a multi-unit bridge, which takes twice the time and requires grinding down perfectly good teeth. In the end, Dr. Fogey walks away with $1,500 for an hour and a half of work. When you compare the two treatments, both the doctor and the patient win out with the implant. When you break it down and subtract overhead and other expenses, it works out that the technology made a much higher profit. Who can argue with that?

You can double and even triple your profits by using technology. Your patients win, too, because they are far more comfortable—both physically and psychologically—and they spend far less time in your chair. If you spent just one day of the week doing implants, you could make upwards of $40,000 in just the afternoon alone.

As a dentist, you are expected to take a certain number of seminars or other educational courses in order to keep up on the latest information in the dental field. Since you have to do it anyway, you might as well spend the money on learning a profitable new treatment: implants, Invisalign, dentures, whitening, etc., the list goes on.

Your charts are chock-full of patients waiting for you to offer new treatment options—the money is on the wall! (We wish it was in the software.)

I have been involved with dental education, such as dental implants and Invisalign treatments. I am a founding member and the technologist for

NAPD (National Association of Dental Professionals). What sets me apart is that I have taken the time to learn a few of the dental procedures—not that I would ever actually perform them, but I wanted to learn so that I could better serve my clients by having a solid understanding of what they do and how they use their tools.

I have also been closely involved with how the business runs.

When a doctor learns a new procedure, he or she needs to offer it to the existing clients first. If you are paperless, we can simply search the database for those patients who qualify, then directly print out mailing labels or e-mail the information. In contrast, if you are not paperless you will be assigning someone to go over charts one by one by hand.

If you are setting up a brand-new office, you can rest assured that I am going to equip it with everything that will bring you up to today's standard of care; all you need to do is attend the seminar on how to perform the treatment.

Renovating an existing office, however, poses different problems, as it is often difficult to convince a doctor that the equipment he has been using all along is no longer on par with the rest of the industry. I hate to be the one to break the news to you, but Windows 98 just is not going to cut it today. We have also found that many older dental offices do not have the appropriate space between their chairs, which makes it a challenge to install the chairside computer or monitor.

Even if the estimate for upgrading makes your hair stand on end, you have to remember the benefits you will reap down the line. You are not throwing your money out the window; you are making an investment that will pay for itself in less than a year.

Let's continue with the implant example. A client of mine from Huntington Beach was gung ho on learning dental implants, but his office needed a complete overhaul. We fully equipped four operatories with new computers and monitors at $2,000 a piece, and installed one set of digital sensors for taking X-rays at $5,500. Add to that the $5,000 he spent on training and you have a total bill of roughly $19,000, which could easily be recouped in a single day.

My client set a goal of doing just one implant a day, so let's be conservative and call that 200 per year. At $3,500 per treatment, that amounts to $700,000 per year. To bring in patients, all the doctor has to do is review medical records and market his new treatment to potential candidates. If he called all his patients who had dentures and told them they'd never again have to use denture adhesive, you can be sure that chair would be filled for months to come. When you consider that that is a conservative estimate of only existing patients and not new ones, you can double that number, which means you could potentially make $1,500,000 from an $18,000 investment—a nearly 100 to 1 return. Even if only **one** in **five** of your patients opted for the treatment, you'd still see a 20 to 1 return of about $350,000.

An older dentist who does not want to bear the burden of learning a new treatment can make upgrading worthwhile by bringing on an associate. Since associates are typically younger, having recently graduated from dental school, the majority have already had some training on placing implants, so the onus of performing the treatment can be on them. To be honest, most younger associates would not even consider working in an office not equipped to perform such a standard procedure, so if you are even considering bringing on an associate, it is imperative that your office is up-to-date. An associate and a doctor usually coexist for a year or two before the associate buys out the doctor, during which time you could be reaping the benefits of profit sharing.

Another common fear doctors have is equipment quickly becoming outdated. We'll help minimize that expense by making a five- to seven-year plan. Let's say we are supplying the computers for your office. We generally stick with our own brand of computers or Dell machines, for which we include a three-year on-site warranty. We anticipate that your fourth and fifth year will also run just fine, but by that time you are running close to needing a technological facelift. That is the lifecycle. Not only will the machine be old in computer years, but new technologies will have come out that your computer will most likely not be able to handle. But in five years you will have made back your $12,000 investment many times over, so that the technology will have paid for itself. That amounts to just $3,000 per year—or one dental implant. Surely that is a worthwhile investment, even if it is not forever.

And it is not just implants where technology can help your practice. Other basic treatments such as fillings can both better the patient's experience and make profits for your practice. Not only were yesterday's fillings an unattractive black that is readily apparent anytime you open your mouth to laugh, but they also contain mercury. Today's fillings are tooth colored and are made of a composite.

Patients are more likely to accept the replacement-filling treatment through the dentist's use of intraoral cameras, which allow the patients to see their teeth in real time, as they are sitting in the chair. They can see the gray of the filling showing through their otherwise white teeth, which makes it easier to convince them to agree to bleaching and a new filling.

Although technology does not help as much in the selling of other cosmetic treatments, such as veneers, you can rest assured that patients judge a practice by its office. By that I mean that it is unlikely that a patient will opt for a purely cosmetic procedure if your office looks stuck in a bygone era. People will not pay for treatment that is more progressive than their surroundings. If the doctor cannot keep her office looking good, how can she be trusted to care for the appearance of her patients' mouths?

There are so many ways to upgrade an office that you need to plan to do a little every few years so that you are not laying out a huge lump sum all at once. A client of mine is preparing to retire, but she has not upgraded her office in twenty-one years. Because she has not maintained the décor or the equipment, she now has to drop a bundle all at once or she will not make much of a profit when she sells her practice. Office maintenance is one of the few times where keeping up with the Joneses is actually a smart investment rather than a foolish trend.

Younger dentists and those looking to move or start a practice need to take many factors into consideration. In some cases, it is actually not worth it to buy an existing practice if the clientele is used to paying old-school prices for old-school treatments. So the doctor must decide if it would make sense to dump all that money into an office remodel if the clientele is not going to be willing to pay for more expensive treatments that will help defray the costs. If not, then perhaps a brand-new office space is the better option.

The other day, I was speaking with a representative from a well-known digital X-ray company who stated that the best way to choose the neighborhood for a high-end, technologically complete practice is to find the one that has the most disposable income. Areas with lower incomes are fine for practices that focus solely on basic treatments, but they typically cannot provide the clientele to support high-end technology. In addition to income, you also have to factor age. True, older clients often require more dental work, but they may not be repeat customers for long. If you are starting a new practice or relocating an existing one, keep in mind the demographics of age and income in the areas you are considering.

In addition to convenience, technology can add a touch of fun to your practice. A client of mine recently upgraded his wall monitors to a larger size so that his patients could watch television, play video games, or even browse the Internet. Other doctors use the monitors to instill a sense of tranquility, such as playing scenes from ocean waves lapping the white-sand shores of Hawaii. It is not just enjoyable for the patient but for the doctor as well. You can never underestimate the pleasure of a new toy.

The bottom line is that technology will not just make your practice more profitable, but it'll also make your everyday job far easier and more efficient. The upsell to the client will be much quicker, and the procedure itself goes more smoothly.

Chapter 5

Customization is Key

Once the decision to upgrade is finalized, I begin the usability portion of my work. This is usually my first opportunity to truly interact with the doctor, either by walking through the blueprints for a new building or an existing office. The purpose of usability is to learn how the doctor and his staff use their tools so that when the time comes for the equipment to be installed, our teams can make sure each piece is placed in the most convenient and strategic location possible.

I will ask the doctor to pretend there is a patient in the chair and to tell me where her eye trains, which can help me decide where to place the monitor. When the patient is prepped, where would the doctor's hand naturally go to reach for an intraoral camera or digital X-ray sensor? Through a series of similar questions, I can get a feel for the best locations to install the keyboard, mouse, monitor, and various other pieces of equipment. This information helps me form the ground level of infrastructure.

From there, I determine where the cables will go; where the power outlets should be installed; and whether or not television, network or computer access are required—which depends on whether the patient's monitor will be used purely for entertainment or if it'll be part of a dual-monitor system. This entire session with the doctor is used to conclude the basic layout of her office and what backup infrastructure is required.

I think of this process as similar to driving that first stake into the ground when you are setting up a tent. Once the stake's in tight, it is a lot of work to change locations, so you want to make sure you plan well.

Contractors we work with know to send us a copy of blueprints for electrical layouts, ceiling plans, and cabinetry plans so that we know how the staff will sit and where their knees will go, where we'll put the computers, or how the new cabinetry will dictate where monitors will be installed. We might look at an electrical plan and see that an outlet will go in the southwest corner, but the cabinetry blueprints would put that outlet out of reach behind a drawer. Such a discovery requires both teams to work together to make the proper adjustments. We take pride in the fact that none of our competitors go to such trouble or have taken the time to develop relationships with the contractors. That has given us a decisive edge on many projects.

Usability is not just about where your hands and tools are positioned. It also covers how you position your body and other required devices, such as the basic equipment found at the front desk. Even the scanner, copier, and fax need a home, which should be in a logical spot that requires the least amount of movement. We look at how many steps it takes to walk from the reception desk to the printer to provide a patient with a receipt. We take into consideration which pieces of equipment are used most often, and make certain those are the ones in closest proximity to the chair, while still providing the employee with desk space. Such decisions affect both efficiency and ergonomics, so we give these matters a great deal of thought.

These may sound like basic questions you would ask a client before undergoing such an enormous installation, but not every company bothers—or knows—to do so. More often than not, an electrician fails to interact with the doctor or review blueprints. We work with some contractors who grumble over sharing plans, but we have been working together for so long that they'll do so, even if it is reluctantly. In the design phase, I like to have every piece of the puzzle—blueprints for electrical, ceiling, flooring, plumbing, even wall treatments—so that I can do my best to foresee any problems that might arise.

It is not only placement that can be an issue. Color can also come into play. During an installation in Rancho Cucamonga, we noticed that the electrician had installed white outlets and switches, so we did the same as well. Unfortunately, we hadn't seen his final product, which turned out to be white rectangular cutouts with a stainless steel frame. Our work looked terrible, so we had to swap it all out. If we had a full set of plans beforehand, we could have anticipated the design and saved ourselves a lot of work. You can be certain I learned my lesson on that one.

Many of my clients have told me that no one has ever asked them to envision how their whole office works together. I cannot tell you how many times I have sat a doctor in a chair and asked her where she expects the keyboard to be, only to be told she had no clue, because she'd never been asked. I ask if she is left- or right-handed, if she'd like it higher or lower, and so on, until she feels comfortable. Most doctors are shocked, because they assumed that there wasn't any choice; they'd just have to live with a standard layout.

Of course, it would be easier for us to do that, but I like to customize design for each client, because it greatly improves his or her experience, both during installation and for years to come. I want each doctor to feel comfortable reaching for where they expect the keyboard or mouse to be, without having to search around in the middle of a treatment. In just under three hours, I can get all the information we need to ensure the setup is as efficient as possible.

Because of their experience with previous contractors, some doctors make assumptions that truly surprise me. For example, a client the other day thought that the one intraoral camera he'd bought to use throughout the office would be difficult to connect and reconnect each time he moved to a new operatory. But I take pride in laying out an office just right, so I explained to him how we'd install additional connectors so that everything would be above the counter and easily accessible to connect or disconnect. That is why we go through usability, so that we can learn how you will use each piece of equipment and corner of your office. We want the patient to be impressed by the doctor's ease with his equipment, as if he has used it as long as he has been driving. We want all futzing eradicated, so that the office works as if it has been choreographed.

Let me share what goes through my mind during a usability session. One of the first issues I notice, no matter what the size of the dental office, is that manufacturers tend to make each one cookie-cutter, with Dr. A's equipment identical to that of Dr. B's, whose equipment is exactly the same as Dr. C's. The result is that I inevitably here the word **"SETTLE"** pass the doctor's lips, because she feels she must settle for her keyboard being here or settle with a monitor there. Sure, that is the way it was designed, but I have learned how to break the rules and customize the experience to each office. Even each operatory might be unique by the time I get through with it.

As I go through the blueprints with the doctor, I might discover that one operatory is used for hygiene, and their hygienist of eighteen years is left-handed. Such information changes the whole scheme. I have seen complete redraws go back to the architect's angle. You do not have to settle for the same office every other dentist has. Forget what the design books tell you; forget that monitors always mount on the upper right-hand corner of the cabinet. If you are left-handed, it *has* to go on the left-hand side. We can and will do everything necessary to make it fit and look the best it can.

Some doctors are incredulous when I tell them that, and it often takes some time to break down the walls that other companies have put up, to let the doctor see possibilities instead of limitations. One of my first goals during the usability session is to get you to see what you desire, not the restrictions the cookie-cutter formula has led you to believe. This is one of those areas that sets me apart, because limitations irk me even more than they do the doctor, since I have more experience with tapping an office's potential.

Once the doctor understands that she is free to speak her wishes, we begin making alterations to each contractor's blueprints, from the designers to the architects to the electricians. What I find humorous is how often we run into the same cookie-cutter approach, no matter how many times we discuss the abundant options. I have gone through usability with some contractors half a dozen times, and they just cannot seem to get out of their rut.

I ask countless questions: How does this space feel? Does it feel right to *you*? Does it feel backwards or upside down? How would *you* like to see it?

Such questioning and realizations take up the greater part of the usability session, since we walk through each area of the office—even the bathrooms. The only areas we usually do not cover are the lab or sterilization areas, although we may point out an ideal location for a telephone or some other small change.

We even discuss the staff lounge. Few doctors give much thought to this room, but you need to consider what you expect your employees to do at lunch, and what they are expecting from you. Will they bring their food each day, or will they go out to lunch? Is it more convenient to provide a kitchenette, where they feel welcome to stay? The answers vary greatly, although the one point most agree on is that we do not want the staff using the office computers for personal reasons, such as checking e-mail or visiting MySpace. This leads the doctor to realize that a special space in the staff lounge for just such a purpose can prevent headaches down the road. We set up a kiosk that resembles a home desk, complete with telephone and computer. Fitting that into an existing blueprint can sometimes be a challenge, but once a doctor understands the benefits, she is fine with the extra work needed to make it happen.

The doctor's office is always a difficult area of discussion. I tend to think that the doctor needs more space than the architect has given her. In some instances, that is virtually impossible. So we next have to look at what the doctor does in her office.

If you talk to a space planner from one of the well-known providers, you will notice that they have been taught that doctors never spend any time in their office, that it is just a place to put their coat before they move to the operatories. Nine times out of ten, however, the doctor needs an office. She needs a place to decompress or to actually perform the work of owning and operating a business. When

I ask doctors what they expect to do in their office, they usually say bookkeeping, reviewing charts, or other general tasks. I want them to understand that unless their staff does these functions for them, they are going to wind up doing it all themselves in a little tiny room. I explain the technology that goes into it, that the doctor needs a much higher-powered computer, because of the diagnostics and charting they need to run. The doctor should have her own printer, scanner, and fax machine, so that private communications—billing, payroll, etc.—stay private. We go through this whole iteration of how she'll use her private office, and almost inevitably there are changes. What started off as a slightly larger version of the staff lounge's computer kiosk becomes a mini command center, with a touch of glamour thrown in for the commander.

I have heard many uses for the doctor's office, but most of the time doctors simply desire a private sanctuary to catch their breath. If you talk to some of the space planners, however, they believe that the doctor's office is a waste of space that could better be used as an additional operatory. But the doctor needs her space. If she is expected to work nonstop with no means of escaping, her efficiency is going to plummet, as will her moods. Some of my clients have outfitted their private offices with full 5.1 surround sound systems and enormous flat screen televisions. At lunch they lock their office door and kick back in a recliner, where they either watch a movie, perform some personal business such as balancing their checkbook, or even nap for an hour—all in the privacy of their personal sanctuary.

One of my clients put over a million dollars into the remodeling of his practice. His private office has a fireplace, recliner, big screen TV with the latest sound system, and a device called VisionArt, a hand-painted piece of artwork that disappears to reveal the television. The doctor is a very hard worker, but he recognizes the need to take much deserved breaks. Sometimes he watches a movie, or he sits in his recliner with a keyboard on his lap, and updates charts on his big screen TV in PIP mode (picture in picture). His office even has its own air-conditioning zone, because he understands that his performance is based upon how he feels.

Then there is yet another doctor in Ladera Ranch, California, who kept the same blueprints for his office that were recommended to him by the architects. I asked him the other day if he wished he had a bigger office. "Yeah," he sighed. He'd been told that the majority of his time would be spent doing dentistry, when in fact he still has to converse with other doctors and perform the functions of any operating business, such as paying bills. When a small group of doctors came to his office for a meeting about business referrals, they could not close the door because of the chairs required for the additional people. "I really shortchanged myself," the doctor confided to me, "and I can't be a professional business advisor in this closet."

I try to prevent buyer's remorse by helping my client early on with what the mini command center needs. Clients will spread their elbows around their desk and realize they need more writing surface or a spot for their audio speakers. The doctor is the captain of the ship, and he or she deserves to have quarters that attest to that rank.

Designers and architects favor a smaller office space because of what they learned in business school: the cost per square foot. An extra 100 square feet in your personal office equates to extra overhead that is not giving back to the business. While that is certainly true, you also have to examine the emotional side. I guarantee that when a doctor invites other doctors in for a meeting, they view him in a much different light than they would if he had an overly conservative office, thanks to the plush leather couches and the welcoming, affluent atmosphere shaped by the sound system and décor.

You don't have to go overboard. The latest sound system and VisionArt are not for everyone. But you do need adequate space and technology, all arranged under proper layout planning. I will admit that the big screen televisions we install do not see much use, but some doctors use them more often than others. That is what I want to discover during usability: just how much you will use different areas and equipment. In this way I can provide you with a customized layout, rather than a cookie-cutter blueprint. Your unique space will better fit you and bring more prestige. But we are also not going to oversell you. If you are not technically savvy, we are not going to sell you on a dual monitor. If you are not big on music, we will not recommend the custom sound system. That is why we hold usability consultations, to understand each office's individual needs.

While the doctor's office may have some flash, we do our best to differentiate between hidden and integrated technology. I have trained my crew especially for this area. If we install a piece of equipment in your office, we are going to do everything we can to minimize its visual negativity. We'll ensure it is mounted a specific way and that the cables are not showing like the innards of some robotic beast. Our use of wires is as minimal as it gets. Our clients prefer wireless keyboards and mice. We can integrate most any technology you want, and you can rest assured that the cables and other visual aspects will either be hidden or nonexistent.

Let's use an operatory as an example. When a patient sits in the chair, the enormous amount of technology surrounding him will be virtually invisible. But when the doctor walks in, she opens a drawer and hits a few buttons, and suddenly the monitor on the wall changes from a serene beach scene to an educational video about the treatment he is about to undergo. That same drawer might also contain the plug to the digital X-ray sensor, or a cabinet might contain the controls they need. Everything is integrated into the environment. Understanding how the doctor uses the operatory space allows us to place the controls and equipment in the most convenient, yet still hidden locations possible.

One area where we spend much our usability session is the consultation room. These rooms need to be sexy, to ooze with success. We would not dream of using old equipment when some of the practice's most important discussions happen here, most notably the high-end sales. All of the technology in the office's other rooms is available here, in all its gleaming, shining glory, because you need to make an impression. You also want to be able to perform any function possible—review of treatment, billing, scheduling—without you or the patient having to leave the room. If you gain the patient's acceptance, you can sign the digital signature tablet on the spot. You do not want to waste your or your patient's time running about the office from computer to printer while your patient waits alone in the consultation room. It is much more impressive and efficient to perform all the necessary tasks right there in front of them.

Usability for the consultation room will cover whether you print out forms or use a signature tablet, where you will keep the equipment for each, and how the treatment coordinator will hand the necessary material to the patient. We cover all angles of the sale to ensure you have the proper equipment and that it is in the most convenient spot possible.

The consultation room is an integral part of the office layout. If you cannot sell your patients while they are in the chair, you need a second chance. That is when you head to the consultation room to educate them on why you are recommending a particular treatment. I believe wholeheartedly in education, both from the doctor's and patient's perspective. A patient will feel much more comfortable when they understand what a treatment entails, and so will be much more willing to agree.

A company called XCPT offers new software that animates treatment plans. If, for example, you want to replace a dead tooth with a crowned implant, the software will animate the entire procedure on the screen. The patient will not only understand the process, but he'll be able to see a before-and-after view of how the appearance of his tooth will be improved. Such technology can make even the hardest sell exceptionally easy.

By using the consultation room, the treatment coordinator can spend the education time with the patient outside of the dental chair, which can then be used for its proper purpose: treatments. If you are spending too much time selling with the patient in the dental chair, you are losing profitable treatment time. You need to get the patient out of the chair so that the next patient can get in and keep the show moving. Do not fall behind because you didn't close the sale. That is the main purpose of the consultation room.

Some practices are still not sold on the necessity of a consultation room, which means they are losing out on the ability to have private, educational time with their patient. An educated patient is one who can make wise choices, and if a treatment is not frivolous, a patient will buy it every time. But sometimes you need that education to explain why you do not feel it is frivolous, especially if the treatment comes with a five-figure price tag. It is not a light decision for a patient to drop $35,000 on his or her mouth, even if much of the cost is covered by insurance.

But if you bring the patient into the consultation room, you can educate them, contact their insurance company, and fill out the necessary authorization forms on the spot. Covering your bases inspires confidence in the patient, and lets them know that they are getting the professional treatment they need.

You simply cannot underestimate the power of the consultation room—or your treatment coordinator. One of my clients just learned that his treatment coordinator, who has been with him for many years, plans to retire in eight months. The doctor is panicking, because he has no idea how to run all the equipment in the consultation room, and he knows that his business depends on the sales that happen in there. When he starts his search for her replacement, he is going to want to be sure that his consultation room has the works, because the first gripe you will get from any treatment coordinator is that they do not have what they need—and what they need is to make their presentation smooth, sexy, and educated.

I can help you with the room and its technology, but it is not going to help you unless you have a treatment coordinator who knows how to use it. Many practices have full-time employees in this position, and they are practically running the show.

Let's say, for example, that a patient is making their next appointment at reception and comments, "The doctor says I need this certain procedure, and I just cannot decide about it." The receptionist could show the patient to the consultation room, where the treatment coordinator can provide further education. But it is not going to work if the proper tools are not there. The doctor's office with a beautiful consultation room and nobody to man it is missing out on sales.

Aside from the treatment coordinator, a consultation room must have educational tools. My personal recommendations are Guru or Casey, because they come preloaded with educational videos and discussions. After the video is over, the patient can ask the coordinator any additional questions.

I want to stress that not enough doctors have a formal education system in their consultation room. They'd rather sketch it on a napkin and say, "This is what we are going to do to you." That just is not going to cut it.

No matter what the outcome in the operatory or consultation room, the last exposure a patient has to your office is the waiting room or lobby—which also happens to have been their first experience, as I mentioned in Chapter 3. We want to make this final impression as smooth and pleasant as possible.

During usability, I ask the doctor how many people will be sitting at reception. That helps me understand the space needed and what the patient is likely to experience. I then walk through the process of the patient leaving. Let's say Pebbles will be sitting at reception, greeting patients and checking them in. She also checks their files, takes payments, prints receipts, accepts signatures — it has all got to be butter smooth.

One of my clients is fastidious about having nothing on the reception countertop. That means the receptionist needs to go into another room to take the receipt from the printer, leaving the patient standing and twiddling his thumbs. If the receptionist has taken the credit card, that makes the patient all the more nervous. The only time we are comfortable having our credit card leave our sight is in a restaurant, so a receptionist taking it to another room can be quite unnerving. You do not ever want to disconnect from the patient, so keeping all the necessary equipment right up front in reception is essential. We'll help minimize the visual impact so that it is as pleasant as possible.

We try to coax our doctors into spending a little extra money on a complete phone system, rather than just a phone. Many clients think that the sound of constantly ringing phones exemplifies a successful, hardworking practice, when in fact it actually unnerves the patients waiting in the lobby. A phone system also comes with hold music and an automated attendant, so that if you are assisting a customer in person, you do not have to ignore them while you answer a call. That is one of my personal pet peeves. How can I, a person who is in your presence, suddenly be of less importance than an unknown entity on the other end of the line? When you've finished assisting me, you can answer the phone. But do not answer the phone in front of me—that is not appropriate.

With an automated attendant, neither patient gets left out. If the receptionist does not answer by the fourth ring, the caller will receive a message offering the options of holding, leaving a message, or speaking to a particular staff member. It is far more pleasant and convenient to hear a live human voice tell you, "Please hold," than to be left hanging in phone limbo before you squeak out a single word. And the patient in the office continues to get the uninterrupted attention he deserves.

For less than $1,000, you can install a top-notch telephone system—we recommend Panasonic—that gives your office an automated attendant, hold music, voicemail, and even contacts the doctor or on-call staff during after-hours emergencies, rather than your having to pay for a separate monthly service. The doctor's contact information remains anonymous, yet patients with an emergency can still contact a medical professional in the evenings, on weekends, or when you are on vacation.

Let's say you are on a cruise and a patient calls with a toothache. The phone system will say, "Dr. Jones is on vacation until August 4. If this is a dental emergency, please press one and you will be connected with the doctor on call." The next thing the patient knows, a live doctor is on the other end of the phone. That makes a huge impression on the patient, since he knows he is still important and has not been abandoned.

Technology does not just let the doctor perform better, or have a more profitable, smoother-running office. It also helps make the patient feel important. With the right technology, you will have a whole new suite of services at your disposal—without having to pay an additional salary.

Chapter 6

Designing The Office: A Treatment Plan for Your Future

When your patients come to you for care, they expect you to provide them with two things: immediate relief from their pain and a plan to prevent that pain from coming back in the future. Let's say a patient comes to your office with a toothache. You first make sure that she is comfortably seated in the operatory and that she feels at ease. Then you listen carefully as she describes her symptoms, and you ask specific questions to make sure that her particular case is clear to you.

Then, of course, you conduct a thorough examination and take X-rays if necessary. Finally, you present her with a diagnosis. Imagine it is a simple cavity. You most likely take some time to explain to her the treatment process before you begin, then you fill the cavity. Your patient is already feeling much better by the time you complete the procedure—but your work does not end with the treatment. Before she leaves the office, you discuss with her the steps she can take in her daily routine that will help prevent a recurrence of cavities.

Not only have you resolved the short-term crisis that brought her to your office, you've equipped her with the information and tools she needs to take charge of her own future well-being. I am willing to bet she is a satisfied patient. And odds are, you've laid the foundation for a lasting relationship with her.

The process of designing your office is not unlike diagnosing and treating a patient's particular condition. We'll sit down together to identify the unique problems your practice is facing and the drawbacks you see in your current setup.

We'll outline changes that will best suit the needs of your clientele, appeal to your taste and vision for your practice, and fit within the parameters of your space and budget. We'll solve the problems that are slowing the progress of your practice in the here and now, but we'll also make allowances in the design for future growth and the incorporation of new technology.

At first glance, it might seem like a stretch to compare designing a dental office to performing a dental treatment. But over the years, I have seen time and again that there is no underestimating the pain and frustration that the doctors I work with feel when they begin to see that their practices are no longer meeting expectations and retaining clients. To make matters worse, the solution—updating the office and getting back on the cutting edge—is not always crystal clear.

My clients often find that after consulting with manufacturer reps, their unique problems haven't been addressed, and so they feel like they are stuck at square one.

If you are working with manufacturers who are used to providing the same design to every customer, you are going to have limited places to turn to for non-biased information about what best suits your practice. And so I have many dentists who come to me saying, "Here is what I want, but I have no idea how to make it happen." They are working with the resources and structures of their particular practices, and they are being offered solutions that do not quite fit. They feel they have to compromise, and in the long run this adds to their frustrations rather than resolving them.

My job, then, is to diagnose the unique problem, develop a solution that starts working right away, *and* ensure that that solution will continue to work for you as your practice grows and changes.

When a patient comes to you with a toothache, she expects individual, lasting care. By the same token, when my clients come to me with the ache of a stagnating practice, I offer a custom-oriented diagnosis.

The immediate result is that you will be able to tell your patients, "I am upgrading the office. Here are the new services I am going to be able to provide, and here is how those services will improve the quality of your healthcare."

In the long term, the design we develop together will allow room for expansion and the incorporation of new technology as it arrives on the scene. My approach to upgrading your office is not just cosmetic, or a quick fix. It is a treatment plan for your future.

Here is an example. I recently worked with a young dentist named Dr. Rothwell. He had purchased his office a few years ago from an older gentleman who clearly hadn't made keeping up with the current trends a priority. Dr. Rothwell quickly realized that while he'd saved money on the initial purchase, he was going to have to invest in bringing the office into the new millennium or face a steadily dwindling client base.

When he called, he was very pleased to tell me that despite the ample room for improvement he saw in his office, he did already have intraoral cameras in every operatory.

His first priority, then, was to get his operatories outfitted with digital X-ray capabilities. It was a great idea—you will remember from Chapter 3 that getting digital X-rays is one of the five most important advancements you should consider for your office right now. I thought we might as well kill two birds with one stone. As long as we were installing computers in each operatory for taking digital X-rays, wouldn't he like to use those computers to take his intraoral pictures digitally?

Dr. Rothwell was on board—but then he showed me his cameras. Unfortunately, they were analog cameras and not set up for digital function. Dr. Rothwell didn't have the budget right then to upgrade all the cameras *and* install the digital X-ray machines he'd been counting on. So I said, "Hey, no problem. Let's take care of the digital X-rays now, but we'll make sure our design leaves room for you to install digital intraoral cameras in a year or two."

As a stopgap, and to give him a taste of our services, we configured his older style analog cameras to save the intraoral images in a digital fashion directly into the practice management system he was currently using (in this case Patterson EagleSoft).

So each analog camera is taking "digital" represented images. As of the writing of this book he has chosen to stay with the analog cameras; he likes the images better with the analog lens versus the newer digital cameras. This is not a failure on our part but rather personal preference by the doctor, and we were still able to bring him forward so that his images are paperless. He is currently evaluating the newest DigiDoc ICON camera, and is awaiting a strong reason to make his choice. I recently spoke with him and reassured him that he must make a move at some point as technology will change. This temporary solution we created will be outmoded, and he does not want to be left behind the upgrade option.

The result for Dr. Rothwell is an office that will never stutter and start in its trajectory into the future. He has the space and electronic capability to seamlessly integrate the latest technology into his practice as soon as it appears on the market or as soon as his budget allows for it, without having to take extra time to move cabinets around or rewire the operatories.

Why reinvent the wheel? If we can prepare for advancements now, we'll save your practice crucial time and money later. It is my job to keep a finger on the pulse of what is next in dental technologies so that I can make recommendations that will keep your office flexible and responsive to the changing times. I stay aware of products even in their early stages of development, so that when I come into a doctor's office, I am not just thinking about what will bring their practice out of the past and into the present, but also what will prepare them for the future as well.

Creating a future-minded design, of course, means that we work with electricians and general contractors so that your office has the capability for the electronics of today and the future. But it is not all about cutting-edge technology and electronics.

I also have to think very carefully about the ergonomics of the office, the nuts and bolts of the design. When I have the luxury of starting an office from scratch, I make sure that the design takes into account, both practically and aesthetically, the equipment that will later go in the space.

This means positioning outlets in locations that maximize the amount of equipment that can be kept chairside, so that it is well within your reach and so that the patient can see his intraoral pictures or X-rays on a conveniently positioned monitor. At the same time, it does not help to overload the patient, or the dentist for that matter, with equipment that clutters the work space and heightens stress. We coordinate the electronics with the operatory's cabinetry so that everything can be both conveniently accessed and easily stowed away. We minimize the number of wires needed to power and connect your technology, and we tuck away all the excess wires that are left over. (We'll talk more about wiring your office in Chapter 7.) It is not just a usability concern; it makes the operatory look like exactly the kind of clean, smoothly-running environment that lets a patient be sure he has chosen a capable doctor.

Wiring an operatory to maximize its efficiency and allow for growth might sound like a hefty task, and it certainly does require considerable care, but sometimes it is something as simple as the location of a door that makes or breaks an operatory's functionality.

Not too long ago, I worked with Dr. Short, who was adding a new operatory to her office. She had a clear idea of how she wanted the operatory to look, and she certainly had good taste. But I wasn't so sure that her idea would translate well from the paper blueprints to the actual space.

I made some adjustments, but she ultimately decided not to use them. Sure enough, when the operatory was finished, Dr. Short discovered that once she leaned the patient's chair back, it blocked her into a corner away from the door. She could not get out of the operatory without sitting the patient back up! Obviously doctors have lots of reasons to come and go during a procedure, especially a lengthy one, but Dr. Short's patients surely weren't going to put up with the chair flipping up and down every few minutes. So what is she doing now? Cutting a door in the wall in exactly the place I had originally recommended.

This kind of expertise is exactly where my work shines. Sometimes I will look at a blueprint prepared by a space planner that looks like it will turn out beautifully.

But when I start to talk to the doctor about what kind of use she wants to get out of the space, what kind of technology is crucial to her practice, the standard design becomes less and less functional.

I once pointed out to a client that though an operatory plan he was considering looked perfectly reasonable on paper, he would actually only have nine inches of space between the dental chair and the cabinet when all was said and done. How would he ever install a chairside monitor?

It might at first seem like an appealing idea to squeeze five operatories into a place where you had originally planned four—five operatories will make more money, right? But when you consider the limitations that a cramped work space will put on your technology, and thus the procedures you are able to offer, you might find that the bottom line is not so clear cut.

It is not just a question of fitting the technology in. There are a number of details that change from doctor to doctor that make a huge difference in the level of comfort of the operatory for you, your patients, and your staff.

Are you right- or left-handed? Are you going to be sitting on the right side of the patient or the left? Where does your assistant stand or sit? Where do you place your lights? Do you need a little more elbow room? Do you need more leg room? Designing the operatory is like playing a game of chess. Everything has to be on hand and easy to access, but there also needs to be enough space to maneuver. Every piece needs to be seamlessly integrated into the whole.

An example of the need for this kind of integration during the space planning and design stage that I see time and again is the practice's storeroom. Many doctors are surprised when I advise them to make a separate space for storage.

You have file cabinets for your patients' charts and cabinets in the operatories for tools—why is an entire storeroom necessary? But do not forget your large equipment! You've probably opted to purchase a zoom for certain procedures, or maybe a mobile surgical procedure cart. You cannot stuff a tripod-mounted light into a chairside cabinet. Make sure that your design includes a room for storing larger items, or you will be tripping over your zoom in the hallway or sharing your office space with it.

So what happens if you are not building a new office, but updating an existing one? Does that mean you are just stuck with what you've got? Thankfully, there are still a lot of options for doctors who are retrofitting an existing office. We are used to working within all kinds of constraints unique to each office and the architecture of the building it is located in, even when we are building from scratch. If your office is already finished, it does not mean you have to sacrifice the usability of the space. Sometimes the solution is as simple as installing slimmer cabinetry. For more extensive upgrades, we might have to bring an electrician on the job, because some older offices simply do not have enough outlets to support the technology of a modern operatory. Some doctors balk at this idea. It sounds daunting and costly, but in fact it is far more cost-effective than doing a patch-up job the first time and having to take on twice as much later. If you put off preparing your office for future updates, you will be spending a lot more money years down the road when you are purchasing new devices *and* rewiring the operatory to support them.

This is the kind of situation my years of experience have taught me to anticipate. I have discovered that the industry has a real need for a service provider who can integrate the roles of the technologist, designer, space planner, electrician, and, of course, the general contractor. You might be used to working with just one of these professionals at a time, and while your partnership might be successful in certain areas, I am sure you've found that there are highly-specialized questions that an electrician or contractor alone simply is not prepared to answer.

An electrician can certainly draw up a functional plot for your office, but he might simply place an outlet in the corner because that is the standard place. If you work in an older office, you are used to making that work because it is the only option.

But if you bring us in to work with the electrician and mark up the plot based on our knowledge of what is actually going to plug into that outlet, the space will suddenly rise to a whole new level of efficiency.

We work with designers, carpenters, and contractors in the same way. Without our advice, the carpenters would have to design your cabinetry based almost solely on the measurements of the space. We can add to their design an awareness of how your technology will fit in and around those cabinets, and how that technology will change over time.

We can also provide a crucial link between their work and the electrician's, so that wiring is integrated with the cabinetry, rather than looping around it and getting stuck under it.

What we do best is technology organization, a specialization that incorporates aspects from the work of the designer, the electrician, and the contractor, and then takes that work a step further. My work is a treatment plan for your future because it goes beyond simply selling you a product to providing you with an ongoing service.

You are not just paying for the cable I am putting in the wall; you are paying for the service and the security of a system that will continue to work for you as your practice expands and evolves.

And, in fact, the system does not just make way for that expansion; it makes it possible. Unlike some service providers who will install materials that you've purchased through other sources, I provide an end to end solution.

Once you hire me, I commit to an ongoing relationship with your practice and the equipment you rely on to serve you, your patients, and your staff. That means that if you have a unique need, I am able to design a solution, provide the components for it, install it, and ultimately support its continuing function. We work together with other designers, electricians, and contractors to make this possible, but our specialized expertise is what will pave the way for the future of your practice.

I am sure you are wondering about your role in this process. How will we work together to apply my expertise to the unique needs of your office? Just as I will design your office for usability, I will present my design in a functional, approachable format. I do not like to work with tiny, 8 ½ by 11 paper blueprints that you cannot read without a magnifying glass.

I work in a digital fashion and keep the blueprints electronically. We can zoom in and out of selected areas and, if need be, print out those areas to share with other trades on the job. We can electronically mark up the prints to reflect whatever changes *your* office requires. I like to lay out my suggestions like an interior designer lays out samples of her work. She might show you swatches so that you get an idea of color and texture. In the same way, I will show you photographs of the new pieces of technology we'll be introducing into your space.

Of course, the most important thing about updating your office is that it will allow you to provide new services to your patients. But the look of the operatory is also enormously important for your patients' comfort and your own. Your personal taste will play a large part in the design process, and so you will need to be able to picture my suggestions clearly.

I once worked with a doctor who wanted to keep all of his operatories completely white, to give the rooms a clean, surgical look. This included all of the technology items such as monitors, TVs, keyboards, and mice.

But once we looked over the pictures together, it dawned on him that white would yellow over time and pick up fingerprints easily. He ended up doing everything in black. That is exactly why I will meet with you with a design book in hand that contains pictures of all of the products I am recommending and options for how you can customize them by size, features, and color. Your equipment has to work for you first and foremost, but you also have to look at it every day, so you might as well make choices that will give you a sense of pride in your practice.

Once we have discussed what you want for your office and looked at the options that will make that goal a reality, I will create a comprehensive proposal, including pricing. I do not quote prices at the first meeting, because I want to allow you time to consider carefully what I have laid out and what it means for your office.

And I have found that if my clients have the opportunity to sit with an idea for a few days, they inevitably come up with questions that didn't pop up right away in the initial interview.

When I return to present my proposal, we'll have more time to tackle those questions and make sure that we have found a solution that addresses your problems specifically. The end result will be a truly custom-oriented design that responds to the particular issues your practice is facing, works within the constraints of your space, fits your budget, and reflects your unique vision for your office.

And what's more, you will have a package that is flexible, able to incorporate new devices as they become available. This is not a system that will become outdated in six month, when the new product line comes out.

This is a system that will progress with the times. We'll solve the problems you are facing now by bringing your practice up-to-date so that you can provide your patients with the kind of superior healthcare they have grown to expect from you. And we'll ensure that you never have to face those problems again by making it easy and convenient for you to maintain a practice that is always in touch with the future of dentistry.

It's important to remember that it's easier and less expensive to install the technology when you are setting up your office than retrofitting your office down the road.

Chapter 7

Getting Wired

You've made the big decision to update your existing dental practice, or build a new one with technological capabilities on the cutting edge of the field. You've called in my team, and together we have designed a unique office that will allow you to provide superior services right now and in the future. Great! With just those crucial first steps, you are already leagues ahead of many of your colleagues. You ordered the best equipment available, and soon you will be able to offer your patients state-of-the-art procedures that were unimaginable just a few short years ago. But first—how do you make it all *work?*

That is actually where the bulk of my job comes in. What sets my work apart from that of other contractors is my specified technological expertise and my forward-minded approach to integrating that technology into your practice. But I am not just going to provide you with abstract ideas; I am going to make those ideas happen. I am here to get my hands dirty. And for a technology expert, getting my hands dirty means getting you wired.

If you've already started consulting with contractors and electricians about your upcoming project, you've probably heard them mention *low voltage contracting*. That is the kind of work I do. In terms of state building codes, electrical work is generally divided into two categories: high voltage and low voltage. A standard electrician, who is certified to work with all levels of voltage, is the one to call when you need a light switch or power outlet put in.

But if you want someone to set up a telephone system, nurse call station, closed-circuit camera system, cable TV, computer network, or anything that involves data signaling, a low voltage electrician is your man.

Standard electricians will be able to put in the wiring for any of these devices, but they generally do not have specified training on the devices themselves. Setting up a computer network involves a lot more than just running cables, and that is where the work of low voltage contractors branches off from standard electricians.

Now that data processing technology has become so diverse and so essential to the operation of any business, low voltage contracting will be a major part of any construction job. Some architects have even started to include two electrical plans on their blueprints. One is the high voltage plan for lights and power, and the other is what's called the *Phone and Courtesy* or *Signaling* plan.

Most of the time, though, architects stick to standard voltage on their blueprints, so we come in and mark them up to include where our data jacks and phone lines will go.

Our process will be dramatically different depending on whether you are building a new office or retrofitting your existing one. The reality is that starting from scratch allows us the most flexibility to create an office that fits you just right.

If we have a chance to install our design before your office drywall is even put in place, it will absolutely ensure two things. First, we'll be able to do the best job possible, because we'll have full access to the space our wires will be running through. When we are worried about damaging your walls or avoiding features in the existing architecture, we sometimes have to compromise elements of our design—though we'll still work hard to find the best possible use of the space.

The second benefit of starting from scratch is even more important: *overprovisioning*. This is my unique method for ensuring that you have what you need for today and that you will be ready for what the market has to offer—and for what your patients are demanding—tomorrow.

Overprovisioning is a staple of my work and one of the prime factors that will set me apart from anyone else you might hire.

When you first begin the process of designing a particular operatory, you might think, "Okay, I am going to plug one computer into the network here, so I will ask the contractors to install one data jack in this space."

But can you imagine an office just a few years down the road where most of the devices plug directly into your network without first filtering through a computer? Believe it or not, this is what the technological world is moving towards—more and more devices that are what we call *network aware*, able to connect directly to the network without an intermediary computer.

You've probably heard of (or purchased) network aware printers that allow your staff to print on the same printer from any computer in your network. Or, you might have a USB hard drive in your office or at home that you are used to moving from computer to computer when you want to transfer files.

With today's technological advancements, however, you can plug that same hard drive technology directly into a network jack, and suddenly it becomes available to every computer on that network simultaneously. Well, this same kind of network capability is no longer just reserved for mainstream, consumer technology. Network aware dental devices are being released every day—it is the natural next step for all USB devices.

If you are working with the latest USB digital sensors or USB cameras or USB *anything*, we can help you set up an office where you are able to plug those devices right into your network drop and retrieve the data they have recorded on any computer in your office. Mainstream technology has moved beyond offices where employees are limited to one computer that can print and one computer that can scan. If the office has a network aware scanner, its capabilities are available to anyone on any computer in the network. If this kind of efficiency is available for standard office equipment, why shouldn't you demand it for your dental equipment?

Imagine being able to retrieve intraoral pictures taken in one operatory from any other operatory, or from your personal office! Better yet, imagine milling a crown from any operatory you choose. You've probably heard of a revolutionary device called the Cerec or E4D – CAD/CAM crown milling system.

Maybe you've even been envying a colleague's mill for a few years now. These machines allow you to take a digitized picture of a spot in your patient's mouth, then use software to design a crown or a tooth that fits that spot precisely. The CAD/CAM system unit then mills the ceramic crown you've designed—right there in your office.

You used to have to ask your patient to wait the customary three weeks while you ordered her crown, and then she had to return for a second appointment to have the crown put in place.

With a CAD/CAM system, when patients choose your practice they are choosing the convenience and comfort of literally watching you mill their crown right in front of them in a matter of minutes.

Now what if you weren't confined to the single operatory where you first installed your mill? The CAD/CAM milling system is now being released in network aware models. You can connect it to your network, and you will be able to send a digitized picture to the machine from any operatory in your practice.

Imagine the earning potential of a practice that is capable of milling crowns for five different patients in five different operatories *at the same time*. I know doctors who are so proud of their systems that they have reserved a space for them to be on display in their main hallway. And why shouldn't they be? We are talking about an expensive piece of equipment that can bring your patients the absolute cutting edge in quality and convenience and enable you to dramatically increase your earning power. My work provides the technology backbone to make this amazing advancement a reality in your office. And the CAD/CAM milling system is only one example of what overprovisioning can make possible in your practice.

The best news is that overprovisioning is not necessarily something that is going to add to the cost of updating your office.

It is an added bonus we are happy to provide as part of our ongoing relationship with your practice. My priority is to get the job done right the first time, and I can do this by anticipating the needs of your office in an evolving industry.

If I had to come back to install a new jack one year after you opened your doors, the cost of running extra cable would be astronomically more than it would have been when the office was in construction and the drywall was open. I am sure the first questions I would hear when a doctor is faced with that inconvenient and costly situation would be, "Why didn't you think of this sooner?" But I am going to make sure you never have to ask that question. I am going to make sure your practice is prepared to integrate any new technology smoothly, quickly, and without interrupting service to your patients.

But overprovisioning is not just something you will reap the benefits of in the future. It will start working for you right now. Getting a network in place that is both reliable and flexible allows us to put a backup system in place that is 100 percent network aware. It allows us to create a high-end backup and data retrieval process through which we provide our support systems. Your security is all in the cable we install.

So now that you know the possibilities that getting your office wired will open up for you, what will the process look like? If you are building a new office, our work will be fully integrated with that of the other contractors and electricians on the job.

We'll be monitoring the overall construction timeline every step of the way so that we always know which trade will be working their magic at which time. We avoid sending our installers out at the wrong time—which could not only set us back, but could also disrupt the flow of work for other trades. For example, if someone is pouring grout for floor tiles, that is a bad time for us to come! So that we can stay on top of these things, we might even be keeping just as close an eye on your job site as you are.

Our work will usually stay right in step with that of the general electricians. What we do dovetails with their jobs. For both the general electricians and us, our key goal is to get in before the drywall, so that we have access to the wall cavity and can make sure that we place our cables exactly where they'll work best for you.

As soon as the wall framing has gone up, we come in to place our cables. The next step in the process will be that the insulation—the soundproofing material—will go into the wall and the drywall will be installed. The drywall closes off access to the wall cavity, so it is crucial that we get our cables in before it goes up.

After the drywall is finished, the electricians will put their outlets in the wall. We'll do our own version of the same: we terminate all the cables that we just pulled in with phone jacks and network jacks. For those working in the other trades on the job, the work is pretty much over at this point.

But not for us. I like to tell doctors that I will be one of the earliest contractors you start working with, and I will be the very last contractor out the door.

I start early, with the design process we went over in Chapters 5 and 6, and then I stick around not only to install my design, but also to get it up and running. Sure, your office looks great now, but what good would that do you if your new computers, monitors, TVs, and cameras weren't functioning? Even after everyone else goes home, I am still there to turn on the power and to ensure that everything runs as it should.

Recently we were contacted by one of our "progressive" clients; he was moving forward adding some new technology in the office. He wanted to place another computer on the back counter by the sterilization area; he also wanted to place a prescription printer there as well. The tone of his voice was, "I know this is going to get me," as we completed his office maybe a year prior. When I arrived he showed me where he wanted these devices. I pulled out my notebook and opened his "chart." Right there was a note about this exact countertop containing measurements to a dead cable (a cable that was placed but never terminated). With the measurement we were able to open the wall and place a standard wall outlet for two additional data jacks.

The doctor simply asked, "How did you know?"

We have many of these types of things where we simply look over what we have to work with and anticipate what might be next or natural. And yes, sometimes we never use the dead lines; it is my gamble.

Sometimes, especially with televisions to be mounted high on a wall, if the office is not ready for the TV—but we know it will be there at some point—we do the same thing, so that there is not just a blank faceplate in the middle of your nice wall.

One of the key elements of any commercial construction job that you will quickly learn about when you start the process of building your new office is the *inspection stop*. All public and private buildings have to meet certain safety standards to be approved for use, and so your project will be inspected at several points during the construction process. These inspection stops are crucial for my team because they help us monitor our progress and provide us with yet another way of keeping pace with the other trades on the job. One of the main reasons why you should be aware of them is that we, and most other contractors, will use them as milestones in our work: a way of gauging how much of the project has been completed and requesting payment for that portion of the work.

The first set of inspections happens after the *roughing in* phase. Roughing in refers to the process of putting all the rough elements of the structure in place—all the framing timbers, the raw plumbing, and the raw cables.

The ends of the plumbing pipes and cables are left sticking out of the floor or walls unfinished, because they cannot be connected to sinks or outlets until the inspector has approved them. The next inspection will approve the drywall. A lot of my clients are surprised to find that drywall needs to be inspected, but, in fact, a faultily installed piece of drywall can be a significant safety risk if it falls off the framing. The inspection after roughing in is a major milestone for our work, but we usually tend to make ourselves scarce during the drywall inspection. It is a crowded time, and we cannot proceed until it is finished, so we clear the way for things to get done efficiently.

There will be a third inspection after the ceiling grid goes into place. Once the inspector gives the go-ahead, the electrician will prepare the ceiling for fluorescent lights, the heating and air-conditioning installers will put in air vents, and we'll run cables for ceiling-mounted TVs, monitors, and speaker systems.

Then the ceiling tiles will go in to close off all that raw material. This is usually a major milestone for all contractors because, just as with closing the walls with drywall, you want to make sure you get the job done right so you do not have to open the ceiling up again.

The last inspection is called simply, *final*. It is the inspection that releases you to move into the building. It is not until after the final is complete that we can actually hook up all your exciting new equipment.

All of your phone lines and network cabling will be in place and ready to go before final, but actually putting out the telephones and computers would be considered moving in too early by the inspectors. Then, of course, we'd have a problem, which means more delays and more money lost for your business. So as a precaution, we wait to even bring equipment into the space until this last milestone is passed.

I have found that it is very important to ensure that the doctors I work with understand that the final inspection is not the end of the project. In fact, even after I receive the okay for move-in from the inspectors, I am not able to begin installing electronic equipment until the air-conditioning has been blowing for two days.

The process of installing drywall leaves a layer of fine particle dust on all the surfaces in the area, including those within air ducts. When the air-conditioning is first turned on, it will create huge plumes of dust so fine that you might not even be able to see them. You do not want to be in the building breathing that dust without a mask, and you certainly do not want it settling on your new equipment. It is so fine that if it gets on a plasma or LCD computer screen, it imbeds itself. It cannot be wiped off, and the technology is destroyed. So you should be prepared for some time to pass between the final inspection and the opening of your fully-equipped new office.

Another thing that some doctors might not realize about inspections is that all work on your project will stop on inspection days. The inspector needs full access to the space and to the prime contractor so that he can go through all the relevant issues and get the work approved.

So do not be alarmed if you come by your site to check on progress and find no one there. We are not out to lunch at 9:00 AM! Check your calendar—it is probably an inspection day.

If the inspection ends early, you can bet we'll get our trucks rolling to the site the same day. Efficiency is always a priority.

One last word about inspection stops. Some contractors, unfortunately, have learned to manipulate the stops to capitalize on the 50-20-20-10 system.

I once saw a contractor play a clever game to this end. He put the wall framing into the suite, and then quickly installed a six-inch band of drywall at the top of the frames so that he could move right ahead and put the ceiling grid in. The doctor he was working for had to unexpectedly cough up a huge chunk of money, because the ceiling grid inspection was a milestone they had previously agreed on. If the contractor had followed the standard process, there would have been much more time before the ceiling inspection. Inevitably, when you take on a project of this nature, you have to be informed about the inspection stops you can expect. Otherwise, you are vulnerable to your contractors abusing the build schedule to leverage more money earlier in the process.

Inspections will not be the only regulation involved in getting your office wired. If you've already spoken to a contractor at any length about building or remodeling your office, you probably know a little bit about permits. Simple cosmetic changes do not require a permit, but you will need one to do any structural work or significant electrical or plumbing work like installing a power outlet or changing the location of a drain line. Sometimes a doctor does choose not to pull permits because he is eager to get the job started, but it is my policy to encourage my clients to follow the right procedure for their city, county, and state codes. If you buy your suite with the intention of building up your practice and selling it, your buyer is going to have to have a disclosure that states that they understand that the entire office was built with no permits. That is going to wreak havoc on their insurance costs, so I am sure you can guess what it'll do to their offer. My motto is: if you think you might need a permit, get one.

So now you have a sense of what the process of wiring your office will look like—what the nuts and bolts of running a cutting-edge practice will require.

We have talked about how I will coordinate my work with the other trades on your job to make sure that I get your office wired the right way the first time.

We have talked about how I will use overprovisioning to make sure that you are ready not just for the equipment you will be using today, but also for equipment that has not even been released yet. And we have gone over the regulations that will shape your build schedule and ensure that your new office is as safe as it is modern. But all of this, as I am sure you are well aware, is only in preparation for the most important part of your project: installing the technology. We'll get to the fun stuff with Chapter 8, "Integrating the New Technology."

Chapter 8

Integrating the New Technology

If you are anything like the majority of my clients, what you are most looking forward to in the process of creating a new office is seeing all your new technology set up and turned on. Of course your architectural design, your cabinetry and chairs, and your office and waiting room furniture are crucial components that distinguish your office, but in this day and age your technology is what will make or break your practice. If you are just starting out, the quality of your technical devices will be critical in attracting and building a client base. And if you are revamping your practice, the technological changes you make are the ones that, above anything else, will energize your earning power. So naturally, the doctors I work with are like kids at a birthday party when it finally comes to bringing their new equipment into the space.

When we start moving you into your office, we will not actually unbox the equipment and plug it in right away. If we took everything out and started hooking it up right off the bat, chances are that you'd see a few changes you'd like to make here and there.

In the least, it is more time consuming and labor intensive to shift heavy equipment around the office. And at the worst, we risk damaging the new devices you've been so eager to start using, or we end up drilling hole after hole into your new drywall while we are looking for the best place to hang a monitor.

As I mentioned in Chapter 6, we try to avoid this scenario by first doing the most thorough job possible in the design phase—marking up blueprints, measuring the available space, and making sure that we understand how you tend to interact with your space and your technology. But even with the best planning, sometimes things just look different in life than we can predict with our drawings.

So I have come up with a method that allows you to make sure that you find exactly the right place for each piece of technology without actually having to move the items themselves around on the countertops or on the walls. I will come in with cardboard squares cut to represent the actual size of each item we are going to install. All of the big features of the operatory—like the cabinets, the chair, and the lights—will be in their static positions and bolted in, so the cardboard squares allow us to decide how best to integrate around them.

These place holders, or props, are easy to shift, and they give you a real feel for exactly where your computers, monitors, cameras, even keyboards will fit. This way, you can be sure you can reach them easily, and your focus can stay on the patient instead of on fumbling for a power switch.

For example, you might have opted to purchase a monitor specifically for the patient to see his intraoral pictures and X-rays during his appointment.

Well, you actually have a number of options for where you can put this monitor and still have it comfortably in the patient's line of sight. It could go on the wall in front of the chair, on a nearby cabinet, on the chair itself, or it could even hang from the ceiling. We will have gone over these options in the design phase, and if you opted for a wall or ceiling mount, my installers might even have reinforced the drywall or ceiling grid based on our best guess of where the monitor might go. But these guesses sometimes change when we are finally able to deal with the real-life operatory. You cannot be absolutely sure until we put up that piece of cardboard and you actually visualize your complete new work space. The final placement might be different from the initial design, but the most important thing is for us to ensure that you are fully satisfied before a screw goes in the wall. The design phase is all about, "What are you going to see?" But the installation focuses on, "What are you going to *touch*?" Where, *specifically*, is your equipment going to function best for you?

There is absolutely no reason to hesitate about asking us to make changes. I'd say that about 80 percent of the time, we find that we have to adjust our initial conception when we get into the actual space. It is my job to make sure that my cable installation is flexible enough to allow for these adjustments. Our blueprints will come very close to what the real space will be like, but every design inevitably involves some fine-tuning. Sometimes doctors change their minds so drastically that I send installers to reroute a few cables. It is just part of the job and to be expected.

Sometimes I have even seen doctors look at all their new cabinetry once it is delivered and decide they cannot stand it. That is a good reason why doctors should go to the showroom themselves, but even then things look different when you see them in the space.

It is not frequent, but it does happen. Some contractors might get flustered by having to make changes, but the fact is that when you are working with a unique design, you cannot anticipate everything, and you've got to be able to roll with the punches.

That is how I am able to offer each and every doctor I work with the best possible outcome for his or her practice.

Now let's not forget that there is a front office as well. You will probably be most involved in the equipment installation process in your operatories and personal office, because that is where you will be spending the lion's share of your time. But the front office also represents a significant portion of the job I am here to do for you. We have got to get computers and other equipment installed at the reception desk, the "good-bye area" (check out), in the waiting area, and—for many practices—in the consultation or business office. The front office is filled with items that are too small to really be factored into the blueprint like monitors, keyboards, printers, credit card machine, and fax machines. But these electronics still need to be mindfully installed so that your support staff can work efficiently.

When you are in the market for a new house, you've probably noticed that the best-designed kitchens create a triangle of functionality between the refrigerator, sink, and stove.

You could not cook if the three of them were cramped in a row, without any counter or floor space between them. But it also wouldn't help for your appliances to be spread so far apart that preparing lunch becomes a long-distance workout. There has to be a happy medium.

The same design concept applies to your front office. We'll work with your reception staff to create a triangle of functionality between the computer, printer, fax machine, and any other equipment that is used repeatedly throughout the day.

Optimizing the space and enhancing productivity and functionality are key. We'll set up the office so that your staff can work smoothly, efficiently—and happily.

Once we have found the best place for each component of your office and operatories, we'll secure everything in place. This means installing hardware to support anything that is wall- or ceiling-mounted. And it means putting grommets in your counters and desktops—holes that we drill into the surfaces and rim with plastic so that you can run your cords between the outlets at the base of the wall and the electronics on top of the counter.

This is the point where you will be glad you had those cardboard squares. I have seen dentists' offices with countertops that look like Swiss cheese, but this will not happen to you. We'll make sure that we do not put grommets in until we find the best place for them. Then we can finally "turn on the lights"—flip the power switches on all those fantastic new devices and get them running.

The most important part of getting your technology off the ground is getting your office *network ready*. That means starting up your network so that it recognizes all of its component devices, including your server and the Internet. Once you are network ready, you are able to print, scan, use the Internet, and perform any other functions using your basic business equipment. Now the only thing left to do is install your practice software on top of your network.

I consider the network to be a carrier; it carries the software that you rely on to operate your practice. Many technicians do not make a distinction between the network and the software on it, but that leads to inaccuracies.

If your practice management software is down, that does not automatically mean that the network is down as well. So I separate the network and software conceptually so that if you have a problem, I can provide a refined, specific solution. Have you ever had this experience?

You order a new computer, and the computer and technician arrive at the same time. Once there, the technician takes the computer out of the box, sets it up, turns it on, then proceeds to sit down and begin to install and configure software. Are you kidding me? Seriously, I have seen this too many times. The process gets more funny when you look back and the technician had the CDs spread all over the place and is reading the installation guide, all while charging you. Later he will be on the phone with Tech Support.

We pride ourselves on being prepared; we receive all equipment in our shop (a controlled environment); we set up, test, and install everything we need IN THE SHOP. Then we deliver to your office. We are assured that the devices have no defects, and we are assured that everything will work immediately.

Additionally, if we need vendor tech support, help is on our dime not yours. Lastly, and most importantly, when we arrive we understand that we are an intrusion to your operation; we want to get in and out as quickly and silently as possible.

Even though your practice management software may be manufactured by Patterson EagleSoft, Schein, Dolphin Management, or a custom software developer, my team is usually the one to perform the actual installation. In the past, these manufacturers installed their own products. We have been working with the products for so long that we have developed our own process, usually based on scheduling.

The doctor wants to get the project moving along, and we step up and provide the installation and integration services. We do this as a seamless partner to the doctor and the project. We have developed a system of trust and mutual reliance with the vendors we support. It benefits us to be involved in setting up your office from beginning to end, so that we can carry our knowledge of your practice forward into our ongoing support role.

And it benefits you because you have one person who represents your total solution. And finally, Patterson EagleSoft and other developers are happy to toss us the ball because it saves them time and personnel. Everyone wins.

So, if you are building a new office and transferring all your old data from your previous office onto your new computers, we'll be able to bring you all the way from network ready to practice management ready without bringing anyone else onto the job.

However, if you are building an entirely new practice that has never treated any patients, the process will be slightly different. We can install EagleSoft, Dentrix, Dolphin Management, or any other practice management solution for you, but we will not actually initialize a fresh database. A practice management trainer, usually a representative of the vendor, will come on-site at that point to walk your reception staff through the use of the product. The trainer will come to your office whether or not your staff is already familiar with the software. The training session has a dual role: in addition to ensuring that your staff is comfortable with all of the features of the program, the trainer will be configuring each element of the database so that your practice is ready to move forward and start accepting patients.

Back in your operatories, we'll also help you with the installation of those two all-important devices we have been talking about since Chapter 3— the intraoral camera and the digital X-ray machine. Being network ready is not just a solution for your computers and other mainstream business technology. In today's world, network readiness extends to your dental devices.

We'll install your cameras and X-ray equipment, install drivers for them on your computers, plug them into the network, and test them to be sure they function. Trainers from the manufacturer will come in to help you learn how to use all of the devices. We are doing the groundwork with the equipment before the manufacturer's trainer comes in; this greatly benefits everyone involved.

Once we have completed the installation of all your new technology—"plugged in" your office—your practice is ready to start accepting patients. After all the planning and execution we have gone through together, you can finally begin to see your new equipment in action. You will notice the difference instantly and undeniably. It is just a simple equation: the better tools you have, the better services you will be able to provide your patients. They'll see it. You will see it, and your practice will grow from it. But that is not the end—in fact, it is only the beginning! We have helped you revolutionize your office capabilities, but we are certainly not going to abandon you to fend for yourself with all this complex, highly evolved equipment.

We have fulfilled our role as contractors once we complete all the processes I discussed in this chapter, but that does not mean our job is done. In fact, I consider what follows to be the most important part of our work. After your office opens its door to patients, we shift from our contracting role to an IT support role.

This part of our job is so crucial that I will devote the next two chapters to laying out its basic components: in Chapter 9 I will talk about our general support role, and in Chapter 10 I will talk about the top-of-the-line backup system I offer my clients. You will find that my version of these services is vastly different from the offerings you might have seen from other IT companies—and I will tell you why our approach will provide you and your patients with an unheard-of standard of security and dependability.

Chapter 9

Fine-Tuning, Training, and Support

At this stage in the game, your office is up and running. Together, we have gone through a very involved and conscientious process of diagnosing the needs of your office, designing a treatment plan to suit those needs, adjusting the plan as we move forward to ensure that it addresses your specific space and practice focus, and, finally, implementing the plan through construction, wiring, and technology installation. Your practice is now buzzing along, attracting, serving and retaining patients like never before.

You shook hands with and said good-bye to all the other contractors long ago, and you've given everyone their final payment. But we are a different kind of contractor. Our specialization is extremely specific in that it zeros in on the tools of the dentistry industry, but it is also uniquely broad-minded in that we have developed a knowledge base that allows us to be of assistance to you throughout the entire lifespan of your practice. You will first get to know us as contractors, but we'll maintain a relationship with you as IT support technicians.

As I am sure you've guessed from the title of this chapter, we move into our support role in three stages: fine-tuning, training, and ongoing support. The first thing we do is fine-tune our installation once we see how it functions when put to the ultimate test: client service. I like to think of this process as similar to an airplane taking off. Of course there is a lot of noise and excitement when the plane first charges down the runway and lifts off the ground, but then there is the gentler, subtler process of its ascent.

The pilot does not sit back and go to sleep when the plane lifts off. He has to pull up the wheels, trim the tabs, get the plane stable and flying a little faster and a little smoother.

Things will be similar in your office. Once our contractor work is done and you've opened your office doors, your practice has "taken off"—you are what I like to call *in production*. You are seeing patients, and if we have done our job right, you are seeing a full load of patients. That is when all the equipment and technology we have put in will be tried and proved, and, naturally, we'll find things that we need to fine-tune. I ask doctors and their staff to put together a *Tech List* during their first few days and weeks of being in production. As you are working, you will notice little things that you do not fully understand about your new devices, or you will start thinking of extra things you'd like to do with your software.

The vast majority of the time, these are questions that do not take you out of the process of your work. Jot them down when you get a chance. After your first few weeks of operation, we'll be in touch with you again to find out what came up on your Tech List.

Then we'll come in to work with you and your staff on each item, so that we can be sure your practice is running smoothly on all levels and you are able to take full advantage of all of the functions of your technology.

The next step is to continue with and to flesh out the training that we—and possibly the representatives from your software providers like Patterson and Schein—began in the integration phase (Chapter 8). Your office is brimming with new devices. These include, of course, complex dental devices like X-ray machines, but they can also be as simple and commonplace as the business equipment in the front office, like your scanners and fax machines. We will make sure that every staff member understands the ins and outs of every machine they might need to use. And we'll train you not only on the basic functions (sending a fax on the fax machine, scanning a document on the scanner), but we'll also be sure that you are aware of each device's lesser known, add-on features that make everyday tasks more simple and efficient.

Let me give you a prime example of the importance of thorough training. I recently built a new office for Dr. Hartnik, who had been in practice for years and had been fairly conscientious about keeping up-to-date on new releases in dental technology. All of his staff members were staying with him through the move, so when it came time for them to settle into the new office, they said, "You know what, we feel totally comfortable with the devices you've set up for us. We are used to them, so we will not take up your time on training." So we congratulated them on opening a gorgeous new office, packed up, and went on our way. The very next day, we got a call from Dr. Hartnik saying, "You know what, we realized we know how everything works, *except* those new chair monitors." We had installed a second chair-mounted monitor in each operatory for the patients, and it turned out that this was a completely new feature to Dr. Hartnik and all of his staff members. Our response was of course, "No problem!" It wasn't something we wanted to try to explain over the phone and risk confusion, so we went back out to the site and gave the entire staff a thorough rundown of operating the new monitors.

As I touched on in Chapter 8, however, we will not actually do training on EagleSoft or other practice management specific software, because the developers of these programs like to send their own representative to familiarize your team with their product.

Doing the training themselves affords them the opportunity to initialize your new database and configure all of its many features to best suit your practice. The training we focus on will be geared toward the devices themselves: your business equipment and the network, the server, and the computers that communicate with all of the dental devices such as digital X-rays, intraoral cameras, and Panorex machines.

Once we have fine-tuned your technology setup and ensured that everyone is fully trained on the devices, we shift into the final phase of our IT role, which will last as long as your practice does: support. As is true of any quality contractor, we place our work under warranty for the first year after installation.

So, for example, if something we have installed falls off the wall, we will assume 100 percent of the responsibility for fixing it. But we go a step further by offering a long-term comprehensive support package that not only covers maintenance of your hardware but also ensures that you will have the help you need if your software malfunctions.

Here is how the software support works. Let's say, for example, that a certain feature in Microsoft Excel just does not seem to work. You will have a username and password that you've created with us, so that you can log onto our system and create an online trouble ticket for your particular problem with Excel.

We will immediately review that trouble ticket and decide whether we need to come on-site to address your problem, or whether we can fix it remotely.

Most of the time, we can solve your problem by logging onto your workstation from our office. We can operate your workstation remotely in real time. That is, you will be sitting at your computer watching one of my technicians—who is sitting many miles away at his own computer—click through items on your desktop.

Or the technician will watch from his computer as you open Excel and attempt to perform the desired function, and he'll be able to diagnose the problem. Oftentimes we'll find that the software is not malfunctioning at all; we just needed to help or remind the staff member of how to use it. Imagine then, the time and money it saves if we can retrain your staff person remotely instead of sending out a service technician to fix a device that is not actually broken.

Time and again I have had doctors tell me what an enormous relief it is to them to know that if something goes wrong, we can log onto their workstation and see, literally and in real time, the exact same screen that the doctor is seeing. Have you ever found yourself on the phone with an IT tech, feeling certain that they haven't understood your problem and are offering advice that does not fit the situation?

Our real-time, remote support eliminates the need for struggling to describe a problem that you might never have encountered before. It is as if we are operating a Strategic Air Command silo—you can rest assured that your equipment is in capable hands, even when we are off-site.

The goal of all my support work is to ensure that you can devote your time and attention fully to what you love—dentistry. My favorite example is Dr. Sheehan. She has been a client of mine for nearly three years, and when we first started working together, she was actually doing all of her own tech support. She is very technologically savvy and is pretty good at fixing her own machines, but once my team came in and updated her office, her practice ballooned so quickly that she simply didn't have the extra time to tinker with her computers.

We originally only worked with her in a contracting capacity, but now that she has so many great, in-demand dentistry capabilities, Dr. Sheehan has signed us on as her official support company so that she can be free to focus on her dentistry. And the fact is that Dr. Sheehan is an exception to the rule—most dentists avoid IT work not just to save time, but also because they have no interest in futzing with computers.

Wouldn't you like to be able to walk into an operatory and simply work with your patient, instead of worrying about the computers, the backups, the wires?

My core goal with my support services is just that: to keep you focused on your dentistry. So how do we ensure that your work does not get interrupted by extraneous technical complications? The answer to this question, and the key to our whole support system, is *monitoring*. We have a system in place that allows us to maintain your entire office environment from off-site. Here is what that process looks like. The first thing we'll do when you engage with us in an IT support agreement is to send a technician to your office to establish a baseline of where your office is technologically.

This tech will essentially triage your entire office: this workstation needs this adjustment, this server needs that update. (Of course, if you are opening a brand-new office, this baseline will be quite different from an older office.) This diagnostic is not about trying to nickel and dime you for services you do not need; in fact, we do not even charge for most software issues. We simply want to get a feel for your office environment. Sometimes we must actually clean the computers with air and vacuums. When was the last time your computer was physically cleaned on the inside?

The tech will bring that baseline back to our office, where we can get started fixing things remotely.

We have invested heavily in our software. We have invested heavily in programmers. Our system will take our input and immediately begin running a series of programs and scripts that will cure or heal your systems. Our software will enforce security policies and alert us or you of anything that needs to be dealt with.

Once we establish a baseline and fix any outlying problems, we go into a monitoring stance. We have a monitoring system that runs 365 days a year, 24 hours a day. We will monitor your entire office during the daytime, and an outside company will monitor *our* office during the evening and weekend hours. When I say *monitoring*, I mean that we are listening to and logging all of the error codes that pop up at your workstation and on your server throughout the day. For example, have you ever had an alert pop up telling you that your printer is running low on toner? That alert—and all others like it, whether they are of low urgency or whether they are emergencies—will be captured and logged by our monitoring system.

Most of the time the alerts do not need to be addressed, but if something major does go wrong, we'll know about it right away—sometimes well in advance of you or your staff.

The majority of IT support companies operate passively, which means that they wait for you to call and tell them there is a problem. We, on the other hand, work in the opposite direction; we *proactively monitor* your environment.

We are constantly querying all intelligent devices in your network (workstations, network printers, the server itself), so that we immediately know when there is a problem, which allows us to fix it without interrupting your work. When we receive minor alerts, like the one alerting you about low toner, we'll usually assume that your staff can handle it, and we will not disturb you.

However, every alert, even minor ones, gets logged. That means that if your receptionist calls me up saying, "Oh no, my mouse stopped working," I can check the log and see that a few days ago an alert popped up reminding her to replace her wireless mouse battery.

So I will ask her to pop a few new batteries in the mouse and try it again, and she'll be back to work in a matter of minutes. If she called a less capable IT company with the same problem, they would have no way of diagnosing the dead battery from afar, so they'd have to send a technician out to your office. It might be three or four hours—and that is an optimistic estimate—before that technician was able to make it on-site. In the meantime, your receptionist has been unable to check patients in and out, schedule appointments, find important contact information in her database—*all day long*. And all for a dead battery.

Now imagine the problems this could cause in a scenario more urgent than a simple mouse malfunction. Imagine if your server were to crash. The fantastic thing about our 24-hour-a-day monitoring is that we'll know there is a problem long before you even begin to see the symptoms. If your server crashes at 2:00 AM on a Wednesday, we will capture that alert. We will check to see if it is serious, and when we see that it is a server failure, we will immediately take appropriate action. Additionally, our system has an "On-Call-List" for non-business hours.

The "On-Call" will jump on the problem. We are licensed, bonded, and insured, and we carry keys to 99 percent of our clients' offices, so that we can get things back on track—even in the middle of the night—and most of the time, you will be able to continue with your day-to-day operations as if nothing happened.

Our monitoring system also allows us to *maintain* your equipment. Most dental offices operate using PCs, which means that they will be receiving automatic software patches or software updates—minor revisions to their programs or bug fixes—all the time. Although there is no reason to be aware of this outside of the IT world, I will clue you into a major element of our software maintenance:

Patch Tuesday. I am sure you've noticed automatic updates from Microsoft popping up on your computer. Well, Microsoft actually releases these updates, or patches, in bulk every Tuesday. Most computers will absorb and integrate these patches automatically, even if you have a very specific, customized machine. Quite often, receiving a general dump of patches on a specialized machine can wreak havoc.

Here is an example. I have had doctors call me up feeling very excited because they updated their version of Microsoft Office from 2003 to 2007. And I tell them, "Hey, that is great—it is an excellent program!" But almost invariably, when I take a look at their machines, I see that they didn't uninstall Microsoft Office 2003—nowhere in the installation instructions for Office 2007 does it remind you to uninstall your previous software. They still have both programs on their machine, so they are using twice as much disk space. Now, imagine if you were getting automatic updates to both versions of Office. All of a sudden, you are quadrupling the efforts of your workstation.

Our maintenance service actually turns off all of those automatic updates for you. You will still get the updates you need to keep your computers up-to-date and running as efficiently as possible, but those updates will come from our core server.

They will be specifically oriented to your office. We belong to a consortium of other IT companies, and every Tuesday when the patches come out, the consortium very quickly reviews them and organizes them into a proper load sequence.

Sometimes when you install an update, you have to take a very specific route, first installing one segment, then deleting some previous information on your machine, then installing the next segment. If you do not follow the sequence, you could end up with jumbled information or redundancies that slow your computer way down. So rather than haphazardly dumping updates—many of them for programs you may not even use—onto your server, we send only the ones that have passed the consortium's approval and are relevant to you.

We are doing software updates all week long, weeding out what is irrelevant to your system and plugging in—through the correct pathway—what will help you operate more smoothly. And the best part is, you do not even need to know it is happening! Most of the time, our clients do not know we have been updating their computers until they see the monthly report. Then they tell me, "Wow, you did all this and didn't interrupt my day?" They are thrilled that they can focus strictly on the dentistry and rest assured that their equipment is not only secured against failure, but *improving* all the time.

Now, all of these features are extremely valuable to your practice, but I will be honest with you: the primary reason I sell my support services is my top-of-the-line disaster recovery system. My support package actually has three components: server support, support for each workstation and the appliances connected to it, and the disaster recovery structure. We can sell you an individual component of this package, but the fact of the matter is that even the best support structure is for naught if you do not couple it with top quality, highly efficient backup and recovery services. Why monitor and maintain your data if you do not have a means of recovering that data if you do have a technological disaster?

When I talk to doctors about this necessity, I like to present it in the same terms you'd use to discuss a problem with a patient. If you show your patient an X-ray and point out to them the exact spot where they have a cavity in a tooth, I am sure that most of them will say, "Okay, there is a problem, let's fix it."

So, I point out the undeniable fact that equipment, even the best and most expensive equipment, does fail, and I show them how I can provide the best means to safeguard their practice from this failure. A server crash does not have to mean that you lose or compromise all of your clients' personal information.

It does not have to mean that you are left hanging, without the tools you need to proceed, in the middle of oral surgery. It does not have to mean that your practice shuts down for days or weeks while you order new equipment and try to recreate patient charts from whatever scraps you can pull together.

In the next chapter, I will tell you about the backup system that will make all this monitoring and maintenance worth your while. It is the same backup solution that a Fortune 500 company would have in place, but because I have been able to develop a partnership with certain providers, I can make this system affordable for small dental practices. This is a solution that is above and beyond what you probably think of as "standard" backup for a dental practice— and I will show you why you absolutely cannot afford to go without it.

Chapter 10

Planning for Disaster and Recovery

"Got backup?"

The word backup has been thrown around so much that it means almost nothing anymore. Everyone wants to know if you have your backup strategies in place. I go from office to office, and I witness horrifying forms of backup. I want to stress here that I do not care about your backup at all—what I care about is your ability to recover from a failure. They are two totally different things. You could have the absolutely most awesome backup system in place, but if you cannot recover from a failure, then your strategies did not work so well. Just as importantly, if you cannot recover without having a significant business impact, then your backup did not work either.

The core of my business is the recovery system I offer. It is a system that was several years in the making, because I spent so much time researching the industry and analyzing what types of backup and recovery systems would provide my clients with the kind of high quality security that was lacking—and desperately needed—in dentistry.

The scary truth is that using an inferior backup system could very well cost your practice $30 to $40,000 each time your server fails. I will show you how this could happen later in this chapter. So, if anything, the system I developed is probably over-analyzed and over-designed, but that enables me to reassure my clients that they are covered in such a way that even the worst technology disaster would cause barely a hiccup in their daily operations.

The key to this is the partnership I have developed with major backup providers who design systems for enormous companies. I bring technology from the big client world into the very small client world, and I am able to offer it at a very good price.

I provide support and service unlike other IT companies, and I am going to show you why this standard shouldn't be exceptional—it should be the standard of care that you should expect!

When I first started out in this business, I was astonished to see how many doctors weren't doing anything whatsoever to back up their data. The dangers of not backing up are obvious: if you have a server failure, all of your information simply disappears into thin air and is irretrievable. Unfortunately, in this day and age a server failure at some point in the lifespan of your practice is inevitable. It is not a question of *if*; it is a question of *when*.

This simple fact has given rise to a common truism in the IT world: backing up data is one of the most desired features in modern technology, and one of the least "properly" used. It's like life insurance. Everyone is vaguely aware that it is necessary, but it is easy to put off—until it is too late.

The most common backup system I see among those dentists who have taken *some* precaution is the USB hard drive method. Sometimes they also use an online backup system like Carbonite or something that Schein offers called eBackUp.

But even though these methods may have been recommended by the developers who sold you your software, they are extremely rudimentary. (And, in fact, now that dental vendors have become familiar with our system, they recommend it hands-down over the traditional USB hard drive swapping or Internet-based methods.)

There are, generally speaking, two different types of backup systems: the file-by-file backup and the block-level backup. Backing up using USB or the Internet falls under the file-by-file umbrella. It means exactly what its name implies: for every file you create (an X-ray, a patient chart, a digital photo), you make one copy of it to store elsewhere, in a "secure" location.

Here is the catch. When you run a file-by-file backup, your server will systematically duplicate each file you have—unless that file is open at the time of the backup.

As your backup device runs down its list of files, it will come to the open file and simply skip it. Now, when you are dealing with servers that have a centralized database, like EagleSoft, Dentrix, or Dolphin Management, this can be disastrous.

Let's say you and all your staff go home at the end of the day, but one of your chairside assistants forgets to log out of the practice management software on his workstation. Your backup will automatically run in the middle of the night, as scheduled, but it skips the *entire practice management package*—essentially all of your critical data—because the software was left open. This happens all the time. But, when you arrive at the office the next day, there will **not** be an error message telling you that the backup didn't take place, because essentially it *did* take place. The server backed up all those non-associated files that happened to be closed, and the system is not intelligent enough to know that the big chunk it skipped was the big chunk you care about.

EagleSoft actually has a built-in feature to help you avoid this problem. Their reps will tell you that every day, the last thing you should do is turn off your database. There is actually an icon on your desktop that says "STOP EagleSoft." And, of course, you have to start it back up again in the morning.

(You'd be surprised how many support calls we get between 7:30 and 8:00 AM from panicked front-office staff saying, "We cannot get into EagleSoft!" And we just say, "Did you click 'Start'?")

But the cold, hard fact is that even with this extra help from EagleSoft, you are relying on each and every one of your staff members to remember to do an extraneous, seemingly nonessential task every single day. There are bound to be slip-ups.

Let's look at an example. My friend Dr. Ward uses a USB file-by-file method to back up his data. At the end of the day, he plugs his USB hard drive into his central computer, copies all his files, and takes the hard drive home with him. One day, Dr. Ward's server dies in the middle of the afternoon. Everyone in the office is cruising along, and suddenly they all lose their network connection at once. Well, once everyone is done scrambling around saying, "What happened? Can you print? Where is my spreadsheet?" Dr. Ward realizes it is a server problem and gets on the phone with his IT company. They tell him not to worry; they'll send someone out as soon as possible to take a look.

In the meantime, Dr. Ward cannot even review his patient charts, let alone take X-rays and pictures, and the IT rep has told him it might be a few hours before a technician makes it out to his office. So the doctor's only choice is to send his patients home, promising to reschedule—as soon as his computers are back online and he can open his calendar. His faithful receptionist is doing her best to alert the rest of the day's appointments that the doctor has had to clear his schedule, but she cannot get into her contact list or her scheduling software, so it is a losing battle.

Well, the IT rep finally arrives and discovers that the problem is a hardware failure. We'll make an optimistic guess and say that it takes him another two days to receive and install the new equipment.

Now he has to reload Dr. Ward's practice management software from scratch. And then he has to layer in the business software, like QuickBooks and Microsoft Office. All this takes him another half day. Finally he says, "Hey, Doc, do you have that USB hard drive with all your files on it?"

Luckily, the doctor does—but the tech still has to spend several hours streaming all that data from the hard drive back onto the server, and he has no idea what the original directory structure of that information was, so it ends up being a bit of a jumbled mess on Dr. Ward's computers. Now the poor guy has been out of production for more than three full days. Finally, on the fourth day, he opens his doors again to some pretty disgruntled patients, and that is when things really get tough. For the next week or so, he starts to realize just how much information was lost between the last time he copied his files to the USB hard drive and the moment his server crashed. That is where the $30 to $40,000 loss factors in. And, unfortunately, it is not a hit that is spread out over a span of time; Dr. Ward loses all that money in a matter of weeks.

Now here is the good news. File-by-file backup is not your only option. Remember I mentioned that there are two types of backup? *Block-level backup* is what I offer—and I think you will agree with me that it is a much better solution.

Every file you store on a hard drive is comprised of many tens of hundreds of thousands of *blocks*. We back up each of these individual pieces of information. The real benefit is that we can do this all the time, again and again, throughout the day because blocks do not have an opened or closed status.

Unlike in a file-by-file system, where you have to wait until close of business and back everything up in one go, we are able to back up your entire practice every 15 minutes all day long, regardless of what files are open on your computers.

When you first contract us as your backup and recovery team, we'll take a master image of your server—that is, make an exact replica of it. Then, every single day you are in business we'll do 15-minute-increment delta backups (which means that we replicate only the blocks that changed within that 15-minute span—*including* those blocks that comprise files you are in the middle of working on). At the end of each day we compile all those delta backups back into a combined image that we use to update your master server image.

The beauty of this system is that we are constantly replicating all of your data without impacting your performance. You do not have to worry about logging out of the system at the end of the day anymore; we are backing up your server regardless of how your employees leave it. Even better than that is the fact that there is no structure to the block system.

When you back up in a file-by-file system, you have to choose exactly which files you want to copy. If you are dealing with a USB hard drive, you have to literally highlight those files and drag them into the USB hard drive folder. So, what happens when your server crashes and you realize, "Oops, I keep overlooking QuickBooks when I back up at the end of the day"? That data is gone. But with a block-level system we have it all, and everything is an absolute maximum of 15 minutes old.

So, what exactly do I mean when I say we are keeping a copy of everything? Where is it all *going*? The first step to creating this fail-safe system is that we install a second server (backup appliance) in your office.

This is the machine that takes those images every 15 minutes. Then, at the end of the day, the backup server recognizes when the network traffic in your office has slowed way down, meaning that everyone has gone home for the day. At that point, it compiles its master image of your server from all of those 15-minute pieces, and it sends that information off-site to four different locations around the United States.

The beauty of these remote locations is that they ensure that your information is highly secure. All of the data that your backup server has been compiling throughout the day is encrypted, so that even if someone stole it physically from your office, or managed to break into the facilities in Maryland or Arizona, they'd only find information in bits and pieces. It would be completely illegible.

The security of my backup system is an absolutely crucial component. You will find that federal regulations are becoming increasingly stringent when it comes to how you are obligated to deal with your patients' confidential information.

Your technology is now required to be in compliance with the Health Insurance Portability and Accountability Act (HIPAA). This simply is not possible with the industry standard, USB hard drive backup method. You are backing up all your files on a portable hard drive at the end of the day and taking it home, so—yes—you are meeting one regulation that requires that you get the data off-site. But that data is not encrypted. What if someone broke into your home and stole the hard drive? Anyone could read the information that is stored on it. And that means it is not HIPAA compliant.

I will give you a worst-case scenario example—and, unfortunately, it is a true story. I knew a doctor who was very diligent about backing up; he actually used the file-by-file tape system, which is virtually obsolete today. One day, he came into his office and all of his computers were gone.

All he had left were the keyboards and monitors; all of his computers, including his backup tapes, had been stolen. He happened to have a backup hard drive at home, but it had been about a week since he'd run a backup on it.

So, he tallied his losses and ordered a new server and all new workstations. It took about five days for everything to come in, so he was already looking at significant losses in addition to the expense of the new machines. When everything was finally set up, he plugged in his USB hard drive, and it was dead. He lost everything. Literally every last scrap of information. It took him well over a year to recover from that loss.

Now, let's be honest. People steal computers from medical and dental offices for one reason and one reason only: identity theft. You are responsible for safeguarding your patients' highly sensitive information: their Social Security numbers, their credit card numbers, and their insurance numbers. If you do not have a system in place to ensure that this information is encrypted and secure, you are in violation of federal regulations.

I have given you a couple of examples of the chaos that ensues when you haven't backed up your practice in an appropriate manner, but now let me tell you what a technological collapse looks like when you've got my system working for you.

Absolute worst-case scenario: your server bursts into flames and melts into the table. Besides your staff members, who have hopefully grabbed the nearest fire extinguisher, we are going to be the first ones to know that this disaster occurred, because of our system of alerts and monitors that I introduced to you in Chapter 9.

We can immediately log into your backup unit, tell it to grab the latest backup (which happened, *at most*, 15 minutes ago) and virtualize a new server for you.

The backup unit will immediately split its functions in half: one half will continue in its backup role, recording those delta images every 15 minutes, and the other half will provide your network with an exact duplicate of the server that just died, so that your office can continue running. All the workstations in your office, your network printers, your X-ray devices, *everything* will connect right back up as if nothing happened, and you can continue with your day.

In the meantime, we have dispatched techs to fix the hardware or software that crashed. Or, if your server really has burst into flames and melted into the table, we have ordered you a new one.

As you are waiting for the new server to come in or the repair to be completed, we keep right along doing software updates and backing up all new information. When the new equipment is ready, we tell the backup server to reimage your new server with its latest information, then we put it in service and the backup server returns to backup mode only. The process is the same even if you have a major theft and both your main server and your backup server are stolen. Because we are also storing all of your data off-site, we can run your network remotely from our servers using your up-to-the-minute, saved information, and you do not have to close shop while you wait for a new server to arrive.

Where once you were faced with a $30 to $40,000 loss because of the limitations of a rudimentary backup process, you are now looking at a loss of virtually $0. At most, if your server experiences an absolutely disastrous hardware failure, you are looking at $5,000 to purchase a new server. And the entire process can occur while you are still seeing patients.

Where previously you would have had to close your doors for four or five days, you can now rest assured that you will never be offline for longer than 15 minutes.

You do not even have to worry about calling anyone in a crisis, because we already know what has happened and we are already taking steps to get you back on track. What's more, our system is entirely testable: at any moment, we can virtualize a new server for you and be sure that it matches your current one. The only way to do this on the USB hard drive system is to drag each file from the device back onto your desktop and do a manual comparison. With my solution, you can verify in a matter of minutes that the process is working as it should.

There may be some of you who are reading this and thinking, "This does not apply to me. I use paper charts, so my patient data is safe from technology failures." Well, the trouble is that there just is not any good way to back up paper short of Xeroxing every last page and paying out of pocket for a storage garage where you can stock dozens, and probably even hundreds, of brimming Bankers Boxes.

I do not know of any dentist's office that has the manpower or the money to spend on an endeavor like that. So, if you are using paper charts and only paper charts, you simply have to recognize that any number of things can happen to paper, and all that valuable information will simply be irretrievable. Do you have a recovery plan in the event of a fire? Or if the sprinkler system activates? In a paper world, you simply cannot recover as easily—or at all—from file loss.

I will devote the next chapter to the many benefits of going paperless, but I will start with a word of warning here. Those federal regulations I have been telling you about will have a serious impact on medical and dental practices that have not shifted into the electronic realm. You are required by law to protect, back up, and be capable of replicating patient data, and so you will find yourself caught between a rock and a hard place if you do not begin to make some allowances for a paperless office environment. I will give you the details in the next chapter, but it is something to mull over here, because electronic backup may not be as irrelevant to you as you think.

My backup solution is all about preparedness. Just as you post a chart on your wall that tells your patients and staff how to escape in the event of a fire, my backup system is centered on planning ahead for disaster and recovery. When you engage us to work with you on backing up your files, we'll help you develop a plan of action.

You can be confident that we'll be with you every step of the way and that because of our monitoring system, we'll be aware of any bumps in the road as soon as you are—or even before you are. But we'll also be sure that you and your staff have clear policies and statements that outline what you expect from them if there is a major system failure. And we'll help you extend this plan to include your obligation to your patients. How will you protect their data? And how will you communicate with them if their data is compromised by theft? By being prepared and getting a tried, tested, and fail-safe system in place, you can move your practice into the future with confidence and optimism, knowing that you—and your patients—are secure.

If you have questions on this topic, I would enjoy speaking with you. My contact information can be found in the back of this book—please feel free to provide me with feedback, disaster stories—or better yet, I'd love to hear about your recovery success.

Chapter 11

Going Paperless

Imagine for a moment that we have gone through the entire process of updating your office, from start to finish. You are standing in the middle of your newly refurbished office, surrounded by gleaming new technology that works at a level of quality and efficiency that was barely imaginable only a few short years ago. You've got a comfortable, welcoming, and stylish waiting room; a front desk stocked with computers and business equipment that make scheduling and information maintenance a piece of cake; each of your operatories is stocked with digital X-ray and camera capabilities.

There are monitors on each chair so that your patients can actively participate in and understand their own dental care like never before. But there is one, tiny thing wrong with the picture. When you turn towards the back of your office, what is the first thing that meets your eye? Row upon row of shelves brimming with charts. Dog-eared charts, yellowing charts, charts with pages spilling out, charts with crossed out misspellings, charts misfiled in the wrong letter of the alphabet. It's like an Alfred Hitchcock movie. How are you going to get out of this mess?

I am going to tell you a little secret that not many doctors realize. It is easy to go paperless. I know—it is hard to believe, but stick with me through this chapter and I will prove it to you. Shifting your office into the paperless world *will* improve your efficiency; it *will* afford you and your patients better protection for your sensitive information; it *will* improve your office work environment, physically and psychologically.

Not only that, but running a paperless office is very soon going to be mandated by the federal government, so the sooner you get in compliance, the better. Making the change will not turn your practice on its head.

On the contrary, paperlessness can be achieved reasonably quickly, thoroughly, and painlessly, and the benefits will begin working for you right away.

So let's talk for a moment about those benefits. Doctors often think of working without paper as largely a question of convenience. And they are absolutely right—although I will show you that there is much more at stake. But let's start with simple convenience. A dental practice that switches to a paperless environment will experience a manifold efficiency increase.

If you think about it, it is a no-brainer. When you need to find a patient's data in a paperless office, all you have to do is type in their name and hit "Enter," and you will instantly see a list of all of their records: their phone number and personal information, the treatments they have received, their X-rays, the date and time of their next appointment— the list goes on!

On the other hand, if you are keeping all that information on paper, you might have their phone number in a Rolodex buried under piles of bills at the receptionist's desk. Their chart might have accidentally gotten stuffed into the Ds when their last name starts with P.

How will you ever know where to look for it?

Or maybe you were reviewing it six months ago, got interrupted by a phone call, and dropped it in a pile on your desk that is now twenty charts deep and covered over by the Sunday paper and the container of take-out food you grabbed for lunch. The fact is that every time you interrupt your dentistry to rifle through piles of charts, even if it is only for a few minutes, you are building up a time debt. It does not look good to your staff, and it does not look good to your patients.

But let's say you are impeccably organized. Every file is tidy and tucked away in exactly the right place, and you never hire a staff member without making absolutely certain that they will guard the order of your office with their lives. Even then, what do you do when a patient moves out of your area and needs their records transferred? Or when you suggest to a young patient that she think about braces? You have to get out the file and run each page through the fax machine one by one, and then a couple of hours later you get a call from the orthodontist saying, "Sorry to bother you, but I can't read page 3."

So, you have to spend money and time copying the chart and mailing it, and in the meantime your patient has to wait to schedule the consultation she needs. What if you could just open an e-mail, click "Attach," and send? You just transferred years of information in one minute!

Now take a look at all of your shelving and cabinetry. I know doctors who had whole walls covered in shelves, and when we took them paperless, they were suddenly looking at cubic yards of new empty storage space. Or, if they didn't need that space to stock equipment and supplies, they were able to sell those shelves, paint the wall, and jazz up the space. Imagine the difference it would make to your front office staff if they worked in an open, airy, well-lit space instead of a dark, cramped storage room where they are constantly interrupted by having to slog through files.

Imagine that young, conscientious assistant who keeps shaking her head over all the trees you are killing congratulating you on going green and getting in step with environmental efforts.

As you start to take your office paperless, you will see an incremental change. Your backlog of charts will get smaller, and smaller, and smaller, until one day—it is gone.

But all of those points deal with abstract resources—space, personnel time. It is easy to shrug your shoulders and say, "I guess I'd be better off, but it is hard to calculate." So, let's look at some numbers. A single DVD can hold approximately 5,000 charts, or more. Most dentists have 600 to 1200 active charts and a couple thousand inactive charts. A doctor who has been in business twenty or thirty years might have a maximum of 5,000 charts. If all that information is in paper form, that doctor is probably spending $300 a month on a storage unit. And that is not the only expense. What does paper mean to your bottom line? Pull that huge accounting binder off the shelf and flip through its hundreds of worn pages. Take a look at all the money that goes into consumable products for your office: paper, pens, envelopes, letterhead, folders, clips, binders, film, ink, monthly labels, yearly labels, rubber stamps. Most of the doctors I work with are astounded to see what a cash drain their filing system is.

You are absolutely right to say that going paperless will cost you. In the beginning you will have to upgrade your technology and train your personnel. But over time, the cost of an inefficient, paper-based office that is constantly chomping up consumable products will vastly outweigh the one-time investment of turning over your data.

In my book, though, the benefit of paperlessness that tops all the rest is the added security. The unprecedented, top-of-the-line backup system I spent all of Chapter 10 discussing with you is of absolutely no use if the majority of your crucial information exists only in print.

Not too long ago, I had a dentist call me up and say, "Let's not waste any more time. Take me paperless." She operates in Southern California, where extremely destructive wildfires had been an undeniable eye-opener to her and many other businesspeople. She simply could not ignore the fragility of paper anymore. Any number of things can destroy your files: a flood, a fire, an earthquake that renders your office impassable. Or a much tinier disaster, like a mouse that takes up residence in one of the boxes in your storage unit.

If you lose a piece of paper for any reason, you have no way of recovering it. It is that simple.

A quick story. A wonderful doctor, thoughtful in every way, decided to have us evaluate his environment from A to Z so that we could assess just what and how to set up his staff to go paperless. We stared at the office with about 600 active charts, and another 300 of on-site storage. After collecting a few patient names, we drove to his storage facility so we could locate their files—just to see the changes in their charting over the years. Once at the facility, I was amazed to see a really nice over-the-top storage facility. His unit was in a building that was climate controlled (he thought that would be best for long-term preservation). When he unlocked his unit, the first thing I noticed was a clipboard with notes of "In versus Out" charts. The second thing I noticed were neatly stacked boxes with clearly labeled information regarding the contents and the estimated year for destruction. What a wonderful job his staff did in putting all of this together.

I jumped right in, completely forgetting the list I brought to locate certain patients.

I immediately tore down a stack of charts so that I could get to the box on the very bottom. With the doctor watching, I opened the chart box on the bottom of the stack and looked inside. Sure enough, the charts were all severely deteriorating.

You see, the bottom box was placed directly on the concrete floor. Over a short time the box leached water from the floor, molding everything in its seeping path. Basically the charts were legible but smelly and covered in mold.

After we shook our heads over that mess, we realized that there were maybe 20 such boxes directly on the floor. Wow, what a loss of information. The staff should have elevated these boxes off the floor on a pallet or even on top of a sheet of plastic—anything but directly on the floor.

Next we got back to the idea of locating those patients we were going to search for. I was most interested in the amount of time per chart it would take us to locate them. In this nicely thought out storage environment, I thought for sure it would be easy, but nothing is perfect. Eventually we found the boxes and began looking through the charts.

I will close with this. A wonderful job done by his staff, with everything almost perfectly in its place, still yielded water damage and mold. And, oh yes, as with any storage facility we found mice, and more than one. They chewed in the side of a box and basically ate the centers out of the folders. It was like looking at chart doughnuts! We stopped right there and then—the doctor saw multiple boxes destroyed but yet he had been so diligent in preservation. His loss was absolutely overwhelming to him. How would he be able to minimize or stop any future loss? More importantly, what could he do prior to bringing more charts to storage?

We did in fact help him get it all back together with a loss of about 250 charts in total, and as of this writing he does not have a storage facility any longer.

We have seen that a paperless office is more efficient, more spacious, greener, cheaper, and more secure, and that is why so many of your colleagues are actually excited about making the change. But if you are still hesitant, it is understandable. I know a lot of dentists who have an almost emotional attachment to their paperwork.

When you develop a system that becomes part of the practice you've loved for years, it is hard to imagine your office changing, and changing in a big way. But here is the reality you are facing: even if the benefits of going paperless do not convince you, the law will. By 2014, you will actually be required by federal regulations to run a paperless operation.

In the last chapter, I briefly mentioned the Health Insurance Portability and Accountability Act (HIPAA), which is significantly changing the measures that medical doctors and dentists are obligated to take to protect their patients' data. There are several more statutes coming down the federal pipes that will further affect health record management (HRM) and Electronic Medical Records (EMR), which will cover dentistry as well. Keep in mind for the near future, all medical doctors and dentists will be required to provide their patients with the means of managing their own personal information. This means that patients must be allowed to update their information electronically from their own homes.

Personal information does not include the nitty gritty of their medical history and chart details, but it does include their basic profile, like their address and phone number, employer information, and insurance information. The only way you can provide this service is to ensure that each and every patient has some sort of electronic version of their records.

The next year to imprint in your memory is 2014. This one represents the big shift. By then, medical and dental practitioners will be required to have electronic records for all of their patients.

This includes X-rays, photographs, treatment histories, medication information, and everything else that pertains to the care you and the doctors before you have provided for each individual who comes into your office. Now, the feds are not trying to disrupt your mission of providing quality care for your patients; they recognize that this is a major shift. So there may be adjustments in the particulars of each law, and the government will provide guidelines for how to ensure that your practice is in compliance.

You can find the most up-to-date information on these regulations on Federal and State Web sites. We will attempt to provide a series of links to help you in locating this information on **www.zlantech.com.**

Now that you've seen the writing on the wall, you have a few choices. You can get in gear now and make the change sooner rather than later, so that by the time 2014 rolls around, paperless operations are second nature to you and your staff. You can wait awhile to be sure that these regulations are really going to happen, and I assure you, they will—and you will be caught in a mad scramble. Or, you could do nothing whatsoever, and face enforcement consequences in just a few short years.

I think you will agree that the first option is ideal, and I want to show you how it will not be half as difficult as you think. When dentists engage my company to take them paperless, I have a Ten Step Plan of Action that I take them through. Each transition is small and close to effortless in relation to the end goal: completely eradicating your need for paperwork and revolutionizing the way you do business.

This step-by-step approach makes the transition as seamless and as noninvasive as possible, so that you and your staff can continue focusing on dentistry, even as your practice operations are radically—but gradually—reorganizing.

Yes, things will be changing and you will be called upon to shift your mindset and some of your day-to-day habits.

But, as all of my clients have found, the recipe for success that I will offer you will ensure that the process will not be in your way at all. And once it is complete, you will be surprised at what an enormous relief it is to clear out all that messy, heavy, inefficient paper and start working in an efficient, eco-friendly, modern atmosphere.

Now, if you want to make the change on your own, I will give you three pointers that will ensure that you do not get caught grinding your gears.

1. ***The necessary technology should already be in place and enabled before you start making the transition to a paperless environment.*** If you are working in an office that will require major technology upgrades before you can go paperless—like purchasing computers with more capable operating systems, software like EagleSoft, Dentrix, and QuickBooks, scanners, digital X-ray machines, and digital cameras—you should get all of these items in place and running smoothly before you start to pitch charts. It is simply too vast an endeavor to do both at the same time, and that is when you will find your dentistry getting interrupted and stalled by time-consuming, frustrating, and extraneous technology issues. Whenever a dentist calls me in to get him working paperlessly and I see that he is lacking some of the necessary tools, I say, "Great, I am on board—here is the list of things we need to

accomplish to make this possible."

2. *You have to have a team approach to going paperless.* The simple fact is that you will need your staff's energy and efforts to help you run a paperless environment. Often, they will be interacting with the technology just as much or more than you will, so it is crucial that they feel comfortable with the change. And even better, if they can get excited about it, the change will happen faster and smoother. Come up with a philosophy that your whole office can get behind. *Why* are you doing this? Is it out of respect for the environment? Is it to comply with laws? Is it to ensure that your staff is not bogged down by inefficiency and mind-numbing tasks? Make sure that your staff sees this as a team effort with team results. We know of a few cases where an office staff member is filing a workman's comp case against the doctor, due to injuries from pulling charts.

3. *Once you cross the line, don't go back.* Going paperless is about shifting habits. If for the last ten or twenty or thirty years, you've been reaching for a piece of paper, jotting down some notes about the patient, and handing it to your assistant to clip into the file, you will probably find yourself still doing that from time to time—even when the file does not exist anymore. Work diligently to break the habit and get used to reaching for the keyboard. If you start going paperless but allow yourself to slip back, you will end up with patient charts that are half-paper, half-electronic—and completely unsearchable and disorganized. Ultimately, this will hurt your productivity much more than it will help. Stay on track. You are making major changes to your structure, so you've got to commit to them.

There are just a few more details I want to make you aware of when it comes to taking your office paperless. Throughout this chapter, we have mainly focused on the nuts and bolts of your dentistry practice, which are charts. But a paperless office operates electronically on all levels, not just patient records. Imagine sitting down to write a letter in a paperless office. You will type it out in Microsoft Word, as you always do. But that is where the parallel ends. This time, you will not reach for a page from your stack of letterhead to pop into the printer.

Instead, you will have on your computer electronic templates of all of your business paper products—letterhead, envelopes, postcards, business cards. You will be able to apply your letterhead template to the letter you've just written and—in an ideal world—create a PDF and e-mail it to the recipient. If the letter cannot be e-mailed, however, you will just click "Print," and your letter and the letterhead template will print together.

Gone are the days of keeping 50,000 pages of letterhead on hand and reordering every six months. Instead, you will simply print on demand. The same is true with everything from envelopes to shipping labels to appointment reminders pages.

Think about everything that can be replaced electronically—the possibilities are endless. I recently visited an orthodontist's office and noticed a tray at their front desk filled with 200 little fliers titled "Care of Your Retainer." They were all set to be handed out to every patient who got a new retainer at their appointment. What happens, though, if the doctor decides to update her instructions or recommends a different cleaning solution? She has to throw out 200 fliers and have 200 more printed. In a paperless office, you'd have that "Care of Your Retainer" flier as an easily-revised template on your computer, and you'd simply click print each time it was needed.

Or how about writing a check? Even if you are already using QuickBooks or a similar accounting program, you probably have a stack of preprinted checks on hand. But some of these providers are currently working on developing a feature that will allow you to create an electronic template of your checks. You will never have to reorder checks again; instead, each time you need one, you will open the template and type in the date, amount, and payee. Then you will print the check on a blank sheet of paper, sign it, and send it on its way.

Paperlessness is not just about charts and monitoring patients; it is about all of your daily business operations. As you move through the next couple of days at the office, be conscious of every time you use a piece of paper. Do you grab a Post-it note, jot a few lines, and send an assistant down the hall with it when you want to communicate a short message to a staff member in another operatory? What if you could send an IM (instant message) over the computer? You will quickly find that taking your office paperless increases efficiency, clarity, and organization in absolutely every imaginable nook and cranny of your practice.

Now, I am the first to admit that sometimes it is just faster to grab the Yellow Pages from the cabinet and look something up. That's fine! You will still have that option. I am not suggesting that you have to destroy every last shred of paper in your office. But I am suggesting that managing business operations and patient records on paper is slowing you down, and ultimately it will be against federal regulations.

So there you have it: a paperless office will make your work easier, and it is the law. There is really no reason to wait. All the technology you need to make the change exists today. We have servers, scanners, EagleSoft, Dentrix, and digital X-rays and cameras.

You do not have to wait for any developments or improvements. And better yet, if you have your technology upgrade in place, there is virtually no cost to going paperless. At the absolute maximum, you will spend $1,000 on a fancy new scanner. So, what could possibly be the drawback? The clock is ticking. Make the change. I guarantee you will be glad you did.

Marketing Note

Please realize that during today's world everyone has an eye on going GREEN. This is a huge opportunity for you and your staff to engage your patient base to let them know you not only care about their personal health but you also care about the earth; therefore, you and your staff are committed to making these changes.

This is seriously a great opportunity for you to gather new information from your patients such as e-mail addresses, cell phone numbers, and anything else to promote electronic communication.

Patient Compliance Note

I recently was working with a doctor who was going paperless; we were seated in the front desk area, when a new patient walked in for his first visit. The receptionist did exactly as she normally does and everything went well until the patient was handed the dreaded clipboard from hell: papers to fill out. The patient was polite but let out a sigh of "bummer." I was working with the doctor on a new tablet computer to be used in the office for the patients to use to fill out their paperwork. I looked at the doctor and said, "We are ready."

The doctor took the tablet to the front desk and handed the tablet to the patient saying, "Please fill out your information on this tablet computer and I'll take back the papers.

You will be the first to use our new system. The patient's words—and I quote—"This is what I was looking for, a forward thinking doctor."

Doctor Resistance

Let's just call him Dr. Tom—a wonderful dentist, about 74 years old. "No way can I work paperlessly," he said. But yet the staff is all for it and came up with this idea that I will share with you. Each morning Dr. Tom is presented with his special clipboard. On this clipboard is a cover sheet of the day's appointments. Behind that is the cover page to each of his patient's charts for the day. This way he can have his paper and make his notes, then the staff will input it into the computer for him. It is working out fabulously. After each appointment he hands the chart cover page with notes to his RDA, who collects them, and each day she puts in the necessary information.

Everyone is happy.

Chapter 12

The Office You Deserve

Remember Dr. Betty Rubble from Chapter 1? The unfortunate dentist out in Bedrock who was stuck years behind the times—and who lost Fred and Wilma's valuable business because of it? Let's imagine for a moment what would happen if she were to pay a visit to her friend and colleague Dr. Buzz Lightyear, who runs an office on the cutting edge of dentistry.

When she walks in the front door of Dr. Lightyear's office, the first thing she sees is a well-lit, airy, stylishly furnished waiting room. In a corner, a mother is relaxing on a plush leather couch, watching the news on the flat screen TV mounted on the wall across from her.

Her two children are quietly putting together a puzzle in a colorful corner of the room stocked with toys and games. An older gentleman is perusing a well-stocked magazine rack.

These are the only patients in the waiting room because, as Dr. Rubble will find out, Dr. Lightyear's top-notch scheduling software and modern, efficient operatory equipment—not to mention his cream-of-the-crop staff—keep him working on time throughout the day.

When Dr. Rubble goes to the front desk to ask the receptionist to let Dr. Lightyear know she has dropped in, she is astonished to see that the front office is equipped with brand-new computers, a copy machine, fax machine, scanner, credit card machine, and printers. The receptionist, who has known Dr. Rubble for years, is excited to point out to her how her new flat screen monitor minimizes glare and makes it easy and comfortable for her to work on her computer all day.

Glad to see his friend, Dr. Lightyear appears and ushers her into the back office. In a nook in the hallway, they pass a new, gleaming milling machine—capable of milling new crowns for patients while they wait in the office.

She peers into one of his operatories and sees a wall lined with impeccably designed cabinets. No tools are out of place, no drawers are stuffed too full to close. Everything is neatly organized, sterile, and attractively displayed. On the wall in front of the chair is a personal monitor for the patient. A second monitor rests on top of a counter just alongside the chair, where Dr. Lightyear can easily reach it to update the patient's chart or operate his digital intraoral camera or digital X-ray machine.

Finally, at the end of the hall they come to Dr. Lightyear's personal office. Again, it is a model of order and professionalism. The doctor's solid oak desk stands facing the door, and in front of it are large, comfortable armchairs where patients can sit for consultations.

The surface of his desk is entirely clear aside from his computer monitor and several framed photographs of his smiling family. There are no charts piled up and spilling their contents all over the desk, no stray X-rays waiting to be filed. In a far corner, Dr. Lightyear has a large personal reading chair positioned across from a wall-mounted TV.

The room is a sanctuary where he can focus on reviewing his patients' cases or invite colleagues in to discuss current research and joint projects.

Dr. Rubble is astounded. All of a sudden, it is clear as day to her why her practice has been struggling and facing a loss of patients over the last several years. If Dr. Lightyear's office is the new standard in the industry, Dr. Rubble can see that her practice is simply subpar. Knowing how comfortable and welcome she feels in this office, she can only imagine what it does to put Dr. Lightyear's many patients at ease the moment they step inside. She can instantly see why his patients are so willing to place their trust in him. If a doctor demands this kind of quality in his surroundings, equipment, and tools and takes full advantage of the latest developments in dental technology, he surely must keep abreast of the best treatments. This is a doctor who takes the care he offers his patients seriously—seriously enough to invest in it.

Naturally, Dr. Rubble wants to follow suit. She cares deeply about the practice she has spent her life building, and she does not want to see it falter.

But more than that, she cares about her patients, and seeing Dr. Lightyear's office has proven to her that the tools are available to help her provide them with a level of care that is crucial to their well-being.

You might identify with Dr. Rubble's situation. Or, you might find you have more in common with Dr. Lightyear. But wherever you fall on the spectrum, it is undeniable that you are working in a field that is defined by its technology. The fact of the matter is that you are running a business, and the way any business sustains itself and hopefully grows is by meeting its customers' needs in the best possible way. Your patients might not think of you as a businessperson, and most of the time you yourself probably think of that role as a distant second to your role as a care provider.

But when your practice starts to struggle, you have to evaluate which areas of your work are no longer meeting your patients' needs.

The vast majority of the time, the shortcomings of my clients' practices have absolutely nothing to do with the dentists themselves or their level of skill.

It is simply a question of technology and the treatments and services that their technology makes possible—or fails to make possible.

The benefits of a technological, state-of-the-art office extend far beyond the care of your patients—though that is a noble and irrefutable starting point. But you will also find that working in a modern environment will vastly improve the quality of staff you are able to attract and their contentedness on the job. If your front office staff is bogged down by a cumbersome and medieval filing system, they are going to get frustrated and productivity will slow down. Worst-case scenario: they'll head to another dentist's office, where the technology works for them, rather than against them. Your hygienists and chairside assistants will benefit enormously, too. When you start training them on new, up-to-the-minute devices, their skill level and pride of accomplishment will skyrocket. A well-trained, highly qualified, *challenged* team is always happier and more efficient than a bored, stagnating staff.

And the buck does not stop with you and your staff. Are you considering bringing an associate on board? You can bet that the young doctors who graduated at the top of their dentistry school classes, who are outgoing and personable, who are brimming with talent and enthusiasm for the field, are going to be flooded with offers from existing dental practices. They can virtually handpick their own positions. And wouldn't you like to be the one they look to, not only as the employer making the best offer, but as a most trusted and knowledgeable mentor? You have a wealth of information and skill to impart, so why not invest it in the best possible apprentice?

Now let's talk about the bottom line. An out-of-date office that cannot offer the services patients are demanding today simply will not grow. There are other dentists out there who *will* offer those services, and they'll be the ones to attract the new patients. And what's more, you could very well risk losing your current clients. Even your most loyal patients will have to hesitate when you tell them, for example, that a new crown will take a few weeks, while your colleague down the street is offering the same thing in half an hour.

But look at the flipside. If your practice stands out as offering the most contemporary treatments possible in the field, treatments that other doctors are only just becoming aware of, you are going to have new patients knocking on your door in droves. And when you offer a comfortable, professional, efficiently-operating atmosphere, you will retain those patients. They'll look forward to coming to see you. And that, of course, means greater job satisfaction and more income for you. It is a win-win situation.

You will not just see an increase in your day-to-day income. You will also be looking at a radically improved selling price when it comes time for you to turn over your practice to that talented, in-demand associate. He or she will not only be paying you for a loyal and happy client base, but also for extremely valuable and coveted dental equipment, top-notch computers and the stellar systems they run, and an office that is beautifully designed and intelligently laid out.

Let's be frank. Updating your office is an investment. You will not be able to put in the bare minimum and come out with a practice at the absolute top of the field.

You will need to be willing to spend money, time, and consideration on this process. But the change will pay for itself many times over. This is an investment in your future, and you will see returns that you never thought possible. Yes, you will make money. But you will also experience more satisfaction and pride in your practice than ever before.

Now, if you are working in a field that is so greatly shaped by its technology, it is safe to bet that today's advancements will become standard tomorrow—and tomorrow will see even more advancements. So, you have to keep a discerning eye on the life cycle of your equipment and on the evolving regulations that apply to the industry. This does not mean you have to think of yourself as a hamster on a wheel, always updating your technology and never getting anywhere. Instead, if you put in careful forethought the first time you build a new office or overhaul your existing office, you will always have room to grow, evolve, and keep up with the times. I can guarantee you that it is incalculably cheaper to make minor adjustments in your technology every few years than it is to do a fundamental, revolutionary update every ten or twenty years.

Quotes to close on

"I run a tight ship, and I have not had to make a change in the last 25 years."

My response to this is simple. It is like watching you put all your money into a retirement account that does not provide you any form of interest, but yet charges you a monthly service fee. You money might be safe but it has not grown, and you have paid to keep it that way.

"My patients will never accept these changes. They will criticize me for the updates and tell me that I am spending their money on frivolous things such as televisions, when instead I should reduce their fees."

I never met a doctor who was really that out of touch with their patients.

"My patients love the decor of the office; it makes them feel at home and comfortable."

In a blind polling of the patients, we asked what they would like to see. An overwhelming response was that the office looked like an over-the-top Cracker Barrel restaurant versus a dental office. (No offense, I love Cracker Barrel, but they don't do dentistry there.) With the results we changed the decor, added technology, and received award-winning praises from the patients—again, in the form of referrals.

I could go on for days, but let's move forward!

The practice you've always dreamed of, the practice your patients need, the practice you deserve is well within your grasp. You can make an office like Dr. Lightyear's a reality for yourself. If you are willing to take the first step, to commit to making an investment of time and capital, it will only be a matter of time before you can pride yourself in being on the cutting edge of your field.

You will be the doctor your patients trust, and the doctor your colleagues look to as the gold standard. I hope this book has given you the information you need to set out confidently—and enthusiastically—on the road to success. If you find that our services match the needs of your business, we are eager to meet you and learn about your practice and your patients. You can learn more about us at your own pace at www.zlantech.com. Or, just pick up the phone and give us a call at (800) 969-3451. I am sure you have questions, and we are ready to provide you with the answers. We look forward to hearing from you.

Chapter 13

To the Future and Beyond

I am a forward thinking person with a forward thinking company. With that in mind, it is my job to stay on top of everything and to challenge the status quo.

We are currently working to move our industry toward a more connected and scaleable environment. We see the growth of the dental marketplace within the ability to "Get Connected" to each other.

Sharing: We are developing new methods for dental offices to work more closely with their referring doctors and specialists.

We are creating secured connectivity for the sharing of chart information and images between the offices.

Scaleability: We are in the final testing of a new method for dental professionals with multiple offices. We are creating centralized appointment scheduling, centralized billing—basically all functions are centralized. However, for serviceability we can take an office off-line. Let's say you sold an office; we can export just the information pertaining to that office. We have a few MSO (Managed Service Organizations) looking at our ability to provide centralization and scaleability for information flow between many offices.

Data security is a top-line item. The ability to keep your data safe, secure, and available is just the most important thing to us. We cannot stress this enough.
We have four areas that we have named as part of our forward thinking approach:

- •DDSConnect
- •DDSProtect
- •DDSSecure
- •DDSVault

Imagine having an office which does not focus on your computer hardware or software but rather focuses on the overall end-user *(your staff)* experiences. An office that functions without fail, without complication, and, most of all, is fully protected from all forms of data damage, corruption, loss, and theft.

As of the writing of this book, we have test environments who have installed minimal computerization, but are experiencing the full effect of futuristic technology interaction. They have no fears of viruses, data theft or loss, and they no longer back up their data. The doctors no longer ask the question, "Can I remotely connect to my office from my home?" You are literally connected from anywhere in the world.

"If you can dream it up, we can make it happen."

I would enjoy speaking with you regarding the future of your environment. Feel free to e-mail me or contact me directly by phone.

PS: Have you "Googled" yourself lately?